The No-Beach, No-Zone, No-Nonsense Weight-Loss Plan

DEDICATION

To the patients whose paths I cross everyday. You inspire me to work that much harder to find some answers.

Ordering

Trade bookstores in the U.S. and Canada please contact:

Publishers Group West
1700 Fourth Street, Berkeley CA 94710
Phone: (800) 788-3123   Fax: (510) 528-3444

Hunter House books are available at bulk discounts for textbook course adoptions; to qualifying community, health-care, and government organizations; and for special promotions and fund-raising. For details please contact:

Special Sales Department
Hunter House Inc., PO Box 2914, Alameda CA 94501-0914
Phone: (510) 865-5282   Fax: (510) 865-4295
E-mail: sales@hunterhouse.com

Individuals can order our books from most bookstores, by calling (800) 266-5592, or from our website at
www.hunterhouse.com

The No-Beach, No-Zone, No-Nonsense Weight-Loss Plan

A POCKET GUIDE TO WHAT WORKS

Jim Johnson, P.T.

Hunter House
PUBLISHERS

Hunter House Inc., Publishers
PO Box 2914
Alameda CA 94501-0914

Library of Congress Cataloging-in-Publication Data

Johnson, Jim, P.T.
The no-beach, no-zone, no-nonsense weight-loss plan : a pocket guide to what works / Jim Johnson.— 1st ed.
p. cm.
Includes bibliographical references.
ISBN 0-89793-449-0   1. Weight loss. I. Title.
RM222.2.J555 2004   613.2'5—dc22   2004017194

Project Credits

Cover Design: Brian Dittmar Graphic Design
Book Production: Hunter House
Copy Editor: Kelley Blewster
Proofreader: John David Marion
Acquisitions Editor: Jeanne Brondino
Editor: Alexandra Mummery
Publishing Assistant: Antonia T. Lee
Publicist: Jillian Steinberger
Foreign Rights Coordinator: Elisabeth Wohofsky
Customer Service Manager: Christina Sverdrup
Order Fulfillment: Washul Lakdhon
Administrator: Theresa Nelson
Computer Support: Peter Eichelberger
Publisher: Kiran S. Rana

Printed and Bound by Transcontinental Printing, Canada

9 8 7 6 5 4 3 2 1   First Edition   05 06 07 08 09

Contents

Preface:
Facts Are Better than Fiction

For a while, I didn't really feel compelled to write another book. I had written two successful books, one on back pain, and the other on knee pain, both based strictly on rock-solid information from scientific journal articles and the results of controlled trials. The books represented my personal efforts to take all my clinical knowledge and endless hours of poring through the literature and put it conveniently into the hands of the average person. Thus, for lack of an exciting subject, I stopped writing.

Time passed. Then one day I was walking through a bookstore when a fitness book caught my eye. It was sitting at the end of the bookshelf, a place reserved for only the best-selling books. As I thumbed through the book, the first thing I noticed was that the author, as near as I could tell, had no medical degree or background.

The book promoted diet and exercise, which I felt was a really good thing. Unfortunately, though, I couldn't find in the book what studies or research the diet plan was based on, or if it had ever been proven to work. Not much better, the exercise plan centered around an interesting yet unproven technique and involved using equipment a lot of people would have to join a gym to use. You could do most of the strength-training part with a simple set of weights at home, the book noted, but in reality, doing the routine as outlined (many sets of the same exercise at different weight increments) would likely leave a person spending half their time busily changing out the plates on the barbells and dumbbells!

Since the book grabbed my attention, I continued reading, searching for a list of supporting references. Unfortunately, it was suspiciously missing. What I did manage to find, though, was a "handy" appendix of numerous testimonials, one of the poorest forms of evidence that something is really effective.

All of this bothered me quite a bit, but that wasn't what *really* got to me. It was the fact that this book, and many others like it that I found in the health and fitness sections, had sold literally *millions* of copies. This told me that getting into shape was obviously very important to a whole lot of people. At that point I thought, "Is this really as good as it gets?"

Then another thought popped into my mind. Maybe these books were helping people anyway, despite their lack of scientific evidence to back up their ideas. I mean, what the heck, as long as they cheered people on to exercise more and eat a little better—they couldn't be all bad, could they?

Unfortunately, I later found out that this is really not the case. Statistics clearly indicate that the incidence of obesity in the United States has been climbing steadily, literally for decades, and shows no signs of stopping. According to the Centers for Disease Control and Prevention (CDC), 64 percent of Americans are currently either overweight or obese.

It would appear, then, that even with millions of copies of fitness books being sold each year and ending up in people's homes, they are in reality far from helping many people at all. If all these books (and all the fitness gadgets, novel workout routines, and fad diets, for that matter) really are as effective as they claim, then why are so many people still getting *fatter*? Shouldn't I be able to find a survey somewhere—*anywhere*—that has been able to detect even a hint of a positive change?

It finally dawned on me that a million people buying a weight-loss book *does not* mean that a million people finished reading it, found the plan practical, and put it to use in their daily schedules. In fact, the only thing it means for sure is that people are searching for answers.

Suddenly, like in a cartoon, it seemed as if a lightbulb lit up over my head. Perhaps with my medical background as a physical therapist and my ability to dig up and understand scientific research, I could make a *real* contribution to what seems to be a problem of epidemic proportions: unhealthy weight gain. Maybe, just maybe, I could gather all the *facts* from the research on losing weight and combine them into a short, easy-to-read book, one that offered "doable" strategies that people could actually put to use in the "real world." After all, from what I could tell, a book like that had yet to be written—a book without the gimmicks or pitches that just tell readers what they want to hear, a book that offers only easy-to-digest facts about how to lose weight. And my promise? Nothing more than straightforward, realistic results that studies had already proven were *really* possible.

What you now hold in your hands is my attempt to do just that. In the pages that follow you will not find any fancy before-and-after color photos of people who have made incredible "super-transformations" in mere weeks.

Nor will you find lengthy testimonials, a list of celebrity endorsements, or guarantees that you will be in as good shape as you were in high school by exercising only ten minutes a day. Sorry, but there are no long-lost, secret workout techniques or sophisticated diet plans either.

What I can bring to you, however, is the following:

- A book on losing weight that is based *entirely* on scientific research from peer-reviewed journals—*without all the medical jargon*

- Diet and exercise (di-an-ex) strategies that ordinary people can do *and that have shown to be effective in numerous controlled trials*

- What the research on people who successfully manage their weight has shown about how these individuals got the weight off *and kept it off over the long run*

So if you want unrealistic weight-loss promises, too-good-to-be-true gimmicks, or a quick fix, then this is *not* your book. If, however, a simple book about practical, research-proven ways to lose weight interests you—then keep reading.

— *Jim Johnson, P.T.*

> **Please note:** I have given my best effort to ensure that this book is entirely based upon scientific evidence and not on intuition, single case reports, opinions of authorities, anecdotal evidence, or unsystematic clinical observations. Where I do offer my opinion in the book, it is directly stated as such.

Acknowledgments

While I may have written this book, it took an entire team of individuals working closely together to make it look as it does in your hands. To that end, I would like to thank every individual at Hunter House who was involved one way or another, be it big or small, in the production of this book. It simply would not have been possible without them. Additionally, I'd like to give a special thanks to Kelley Blewster, Alexandra Mummery, Jeanne Brondino, and Kiran Rana for their key roles.

I would also like to thank my dad, one of my real-life heroes, for always giving me good advice, and my mom for just being the best mom I could ask for. Not enough can be said for giving a child a good foundation to grow on, and in that I feel they succeeded.

And last but not least, I owe yet another big "thank you" to my wife, Cathy. It's true that behind every good man there is a good woman. In this case, she was usually doing the laundry, cooking dinner, and helping the kids with their homework so that I could have the luxury of writing this book.

IMPORTANT NOTE

1

Save Yourself Some Time— Know These Basics *Before* You Begin

When you're armed with the facts, your journey becomes easier

As I remember, it was about two in the afternoon that day. Through its twists and turns, life had led me to a gross-anatomy class where I was put into a small group and assigned to a cadaver, a human corpse that is cut apart for scientific examination. I had beaten out stiff competition to get into physical-therapy school—some four hundred–plus applicants for a mere thirty-eight slots—but today I would have traded places with any of them.

The instructor told us to begin. We all stood there quietly, just staring at the cadaver lying face up on the table, nobody really wanting to make the first cut with their scalpel. After what seemed like a lifetime, someone finally spoke up and said, "Alright, I'll do it."

The rest of us just watched (well, most of us anyway) as the action began and the skin separated, instantly revealing a yellowish substance underneath. It was a fine layer of fat, or what I later learned to call *adipose tissue*.

HERE'S WHAT THE FUSS IS ALL ABOUT

I have yet to pick up a book on weight loss that gives the reader a basic understanding of the very problem it's trying to tackle: fat! As I see it, the more you know about this annoying little substance, such as what its purpose is and how it works, the more successful you're going to be at getting rid of it. It's kind of like that old Chinese proverb—you know, the one that goes "Know thine enemy."

Doctors call fat *adipose* or *adipose tissue*. The story of your adipose tissue began some time ago when you were only in your second trimester of life, still in your mother's uterus. It was around then that fat cells, known as *adipocytes* (that's pronounced add-i-poh-sites), began to form.

By the time you were fully grown, you probably ended up with somewhere around thirty to thirty-five billion of these adipocytes. Highly controversial, however, is the question of whether the number of adipocytes you have as an adult remains the same, or if it can actually increase. According to the latest research, the jury's still out on this one.

If you reach down and pinch a little bit of fat from around your stomach area, the following picture (Figure 1.1) is a close-up look at what the fat, or adipocytes, that you hold between your fingers looks like:

They sort of look like tiny balloons, don't they? As a matter of fact, they work a lot like balloons too. You see, if you happen to eat more food than you need on a given day, your body says, "Hey, I don't need all this food right now, so I'd better save it for when it might come in handy." And so your body efficiently converts what you don't need into fat

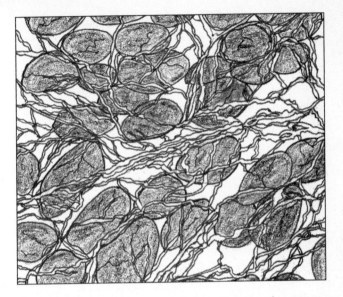

Figure 1.1. From the human abdomen. Drawing of a scanning electron micrograph showing human adipocytes covered by strands of connective tissue.

and stuffs the fat into (you guessed it) the adipocyte cell. It's all basically a survival kind of thing and really comes in quite handy. For instance, just think of the last time you were sick and didn't really feel like eating very much. You can thank the stored fat in your adipocytes for keeping your body running until you got back on your feet.

Normally, fat makes up about 10 percent of your total body weight, giving you about a forty-day backup supply of energy—and that's definitely a good thing. The downside, however, is that these adipocytes, just like balloons, can "blow up" and hold an amazing amount of fat. Therefore, the more surplus food you eat, the more surplus fat your body has to stuff into your fat cells to save for a rainy day. Problem is, the bigger the fat cells get, the bigger *you* get.

Don't get too discouraged, though, because the whole process described above can also be reversed—if you know how. The trick is to make your body *want* to take the fat out of the adipocyte, which it will be more than happy to do when it runs out of energy. Question is, how do we make your body run low on energy?

There are two good ways. You can either give your body a smaller supply of energy to run on than it needs (a diet strategy) *or* you can burn up more energy than you've given it that day (an exercise strategy). Using either one of these two strategies, or preferably both, forces your body to reach into your adipocytes to get some fat for energy. This, of course, makes the adipocytes smaller, and the smaller they get, the better you look in the mirror. As you can see, losing weight in principle is really no different from letting the air out of a balloon. It's finding the easiest and most effective way to "let the air out" that becomes the hard part.

The last thing you will want to know about these adipocytes is that as you get thinner, your fat cells never disappear; rather, they just shrink in size. The only way to actually get rid of the fat cell itself is to physically remove it, liposuction being one such method.

THE TRUTH ABOUT CELLULITE

Just about everyone has heard the word *cellulite*, usually from women who are talking about that lovely "orange peel" or "cottage cheese" appearance frequently seen on their thigh and buttock areas. Since there seems to be a lot of mystery and misunderstanding going around about this cellulite stuff, let's just stick to some of the known medical facts (Rosenbaum, 1998):

◆ The layer of connective tissue that is right below the skin has a more irregular and broken-up pattern in people who have cellulite.

◆ Fat pushing up into this irregular pattern of connective tissue causes the familiar dimpling effect that you see.

◆ This irregular pattern of connective tissue is much more common in females, which explains why cellulite is mainly seen in women. The same layer of connective tissue in men is usually smooth and continuous.

◆ Interestingly, studies of men who *do* have cellulite show that they have the same irregular connective-tissue patterns as females.

◆ Cellulite can affect someone whether they are overweight or not, because the main reason for it is the irregular pattern of the connective tissue. Excess weight, however, does makes it more visible.

It would appear, then, that cellulite is really nothing more than just your run-of-the-mill kind of fat. The real culprit seems to be an irregular pattern of connective tissue that lies right beneath the skin and gives ordinary fat the ability to bulge out and change the appearance of your hips and thighs. While the stuff may look awful, it is good to know that it isn't harmful in the least.

Losing weight *can* have some effect on cellulite because it effectively shrinks the fat cells that are pushing up on the skin and causing it to dimple. However, losing weight may not be enough to totally get rid of the cellulite "look" (remember, cellulite can be seen in thin women as well), because losing weight does not physically change the underlying structure of your connective tissue. Therefore, to really eliminate cellulite, one would have to use a treatment that somehow changes the irregular pattern of tissue under the skin.

WHAT YOU NEED TO KNOW ABOUT SPOT REDUCING

While we're discussing hot weight-loss topics, we might as well cover one of the biggest of them all: spot reduction. For some reason, probably based less on reason and more on hope, there is a widely held opinion that you can selectively reduce the amount of fat over a particular part of the body by exercising it. Believers in this theory, for instance, do sit-ups to lose stomach fat or leg raises to get rid of thigh fat. If you think about it, there is a bit of logic to it. But what's the *real* story?

The answer to this question lies in the results of several studies, such as one conducted at the University of Massachusetts twenty years ago (Katch, 1984). Researchers had a group of subjects do over five thousand sit-ups in a twenty-seven-day period. Changes in the size of fat cells and body composition were checked before and after the study and compared to those of a control group that did not exercise. The results? Sit-ups *did not* selectively reduce the size of the fat cells in the stomach or significantly change the thickness of the abdominal layer of fat.

Other, less complicated studies have also reached the same conclusions. For example, one looked at the size and fat thickness of the arms of tennis players (Gwinup, 1971). The thinking here was that if spot reduction really worked, then the "working" arm of tennis players should have a lot less fat on it than their other, "inactive" arm. Once again, the theory of spot reducing was not supported, as *no* significant differences were found in the thickness of fat over the muscles of the players' racquet arm, the one clearly getting more exercise.

In light of the research, the real story about spot reduction is that this most appealing idea is clearly just a myth. One of the best ways of getting rid of body fat in certain areas is by making your body reach into that fat cell for reserve energy by using diet and exercise strategies. Over time, *many* different areas on your body where you store fat will get smaller—which will more than likely include the area you want to reduce the most!

HOW TO TELL IF YOUR WEIGHT IS PUTTING YOUR HEALTH AT RISK

Of course you know that putting on too many extra pounds is a bad thing; *everyone* knows that. It's here that we need to take the discussion a step further. What we really need to know is *how much* extra fat is too much and at what point it starts putting our health at risk.

In order to get answers to these questions, we first need a good way to determine just how much total body fat we're actually carrying around. Some of the best methods for figuring this out include total body water, total body potassium, bioelectrical impedance, and dual-energy X-ray absorptiometry.

I already know what you're thinking: Yeah, right. While

it is true that these are all good methods, they are often expensive and not very practical for you or me to use on a regular basis. That's why the next best thing is what is known as the *body mass index*, or BMI for short. While the BMI does not directly measure fat, it succeeds quite nicely in giving each of us a number that *does* significantly correlate with our total body-fat content. You also might be interested to know that the CDC, Surgeon General, and the National Institutes of Health all promote and endorse the use of the BMI. The following are some very good reasons why just about everyone likes to use the BMI:

- ◆ It's simple, rapid, and inexpensive.

- ◆ It's a more accurate measure of total body fat than relying on weight alone.

- ◆ It works for adult men, adult nonpregnant women, and generally all racial/ethnic groups.

- ◆ It is more highly correlated with body fat than any other indicator of height and weight.

- ◆ It has been shown to correlate with a person's risk of health problems. As an example, your risk of getting heart disease increases as your BMI number increases above a certain range.

As you can see, the BMI is a very useful and well-researched tool. To find out what your BMI is, grab any simple calculator and follow these three easy steps:

1. Multiply your weight in pounds by 705.

2. Divide your answer by your height in inches.

3. Now divide this answer by your height in inches again.

The result is your BMI.

Pretty easy, huh? Now here's a real-life example to make sure you're on the right track.

Let's say that you are 5' 6" (66 inches) and you weigh 185 pounds:

185 multiplied by 705 = 130,425

130,425 divided by 66 = 1,976.14

1,976.14 divided by 66 = 29.94, or a BMI of 29.9

Okay, enough math. Now that you've got your own personal BMI number, what does it *really* mean? Well first of all, researchers use the BMI number to classify people into different weight categories. So, according to the experts, this is how the cookie crumbles:

If your BMI is below 18.5...   you're underweight

If your BMI is 18.5 to 24.9...   you're in the "ideal" range

If your BMI is 25 to 29.9...   you're overweight

If your BMI is 30 or higher...   you're obese

With your BMI number and the above list, you will now be able to look at your weight the same way doctors and dieticians do. Know also that the BMI does have a few limitations. It may *overestimate* body fat if you are pretty muscular (such as a bodybuilder), or it can even *underestimate* body fat if you have lost a lot of muscle mass (like an elderly person). Also, it may not be accurate for persons under five feet tall. Having said that, the BMI still remains a widely recommended and widely used tool by researchers and health professionals alike.

Using the very same classification system as the one above, researchers have taken large groups of people, determined their BMI numbers, and then looked closely at any health problems they might have. What the research has shown us (Stunkard, 1993; NIH, 1998) is that if you have a BMI of 25 or above, you are at increased risk for such problems as

- high blood pressure
- type-2 diabetes (non–insulin dependent)
- heart disease
- depression
- high cholesterol
- congestive heart failure
- osteoarthritis
- gout
- gallstones
- stroke
- sleep apnea
- colon cancer
- cancer of the gallbladder
- breast cancer
- endometrial cancer
- menstrual irregularities

Quite a lengthy list, isn't it? It appears that besides changing the way you look, carrying around a certain

amount of extra fat can have a lot of serious health consequences as well. Know too, though, that having a BMI of 25
or above *does not necessarily* mean that you are unhealthy
or will for certain get any or all of these health problems.
This is because the BMI is not diagnostic in and of itself,
but is rather just one of *many* risk factors that are used to
predict your risk of getting a disease. Others that might enter into the overall picture include things such as your fam-
ily medical history and habits such as smoking.

The main thing you need to be aware of is that there are
many variables that need to be taken into account when
deciding how likely it is that you will a get a health problem, but having a BMI of 25 or above is one of those important variables. This is because many studies have
pointed out that as your BMI number increases above a
certain range, so does your risk of getting many diseases.

IF YOU CARRY YOUR WEIGHT HERE, YOU COULD BE HEADED FOR TROUBLE

Have you ever seen a person with a huge, plump belly? Of
course you have. How about a person with fat eyelids? Fat
ears? Probably never. From these simple observations, it's
quite clear that there are some places where Mother Nature
has chosen to put fat, while others appear to be off-limits.
Although this observation may seem rather trivial, there's
really more here than meets the eye.

You have learned that high BMI numbers are linked to
certain ailments. What you probably don't know, however,
is that *where* you carry around this added weight also makes
a mighty big difference when it comes to your health.

If you have a tendency to carry your fat on your upper body, waist, and abdomen, then you have what is sometimes called an "apple shape." On the other hand, if you lean more towards putting fat on your lower body, hips, and thighs, then you are more of a "pear shape." To make a long story short, "apples" tend to have more health problems than "pears" do (Pi-Sunyer, 1999).

We know this to be true because researchers, noticing these body types, began actively studying the following two particular areas of the body where people commonly store their fat:

1. the abdominal or "stomach area" and

2. the thigh or "upper leg area"

Just as with the BMI, researchers have analyzed large groups of people. After looking at both their health *and* where they carry their fat, it was found that people who store their fat more "centrally"—that is, in their upper body and stomach area (the apples)—were more at risk for

◆ high blood pressure

◆ diabetes, type 2

◆ heart disease

◆ stroke

At this point, you are probably wondering if you are carrying too much fat around your stomach area and are at risk for getting these nasty health problems. Well don't worry, I won't leave you guessing.

One of the best rough-and-ready ways to determine if your "central," or stomach, fat is a hazard to your health is to measure your waist. People in the weight-loss field call

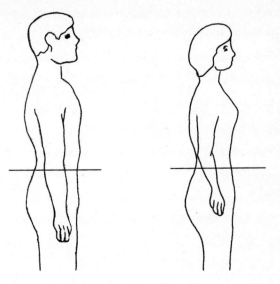

Figure 1.2. Measuring your waist circumference

this your *waist circumference*. It's well researched, done quickly, and very practical—making it our tool of choice.

Measuring your waist circumference is easy. All you need is a tape measure that will go around your waist. Ready? Here's what to do:

- First, find your hip bone on one side (it is located below the line in Figure 1.2).

- Place your tape measure just above this bone. This will be exactly where the lines are located in the above pictures.

- The tape measure should be parallel (level) with the floor.

- The tape measure should be pulled snug, not tight.

◆ Take the measurement as you are quietly and normally breathing.

You now have your very own waist-circumference measurement, which does a good job of assessing your abdominal-fat content. If either of the following statements applies to you, you are at risk for the health problems I mentioned earlier in this section:

◆ if you are a man and your waist measures more than 40 inches

or

◆ if you are a woman and your waist measures more than 35 inches

These waist-circumference end points (40 inches for men and 35 inches for women) can generally be used by all adults. Like any test, however, using waist circumference also has its limitations. If you are under five feet tall or your BMI number is 35 or higher, these end points may not apply.

WHY YOUR WEIGHT PROBLEM ISN'T ALL YOUR FAULT

A lot of people are motivated to lose weight because they don't like the way they look in the mirror. After reading about the health risks associated with weighing too much, you are now keenly aware of more good reasons to slim down, such as lowering your risk of diabetes, stroke, certain types of cancer, and heart disease.

Although these are all very serious consequences of having too much extra fat, and although they put your health at risk, it also needs to be said that you shouldn't be too hard on yourself for being in this situation.

In his book *The Way to Eat*, Dr. David Katz, a professor at Yale University School of Medicine, compares us to polar bears in the desert. Polar bears are designed to live in very cold climates and are very efficient at conserving heat—nothing at all wrong with that; that's how they're supposed to work. However, if you were to stick polar bears in the middle of a hot desert, the very same thing that kept them alive in a cold climate (being good at conserving heat) would now work *against* them and threaten their very survival.

People today are in a similar predicament. A long time ago, human beings had to hunt down their dinner and rely upon wild-growing plants and such. Food was far from being readily available. This situation helps explain why our bodies are so good at storing extra energy and why we have a tendency to overeat when food is around—it's a survival mechanism of sorts. But, just like the polar bear's ability to conserve heat would get him in a lot of trouble in the hot desert, our survival mechanism is now also working against us. Our bodies are very efficient at storing extra food because we needed to be able to do that thousands of years ago, but put us in an environment of super-size portions, fast foods, and vending machines and, well, you can see what the result is—the epidemic of unhealthy weight levels we have on our hands today! It is my opinion that you can blame yourself only so much for things like overeating, because we're really just doing what we have a natural tendency to do. Unfortunately, we have these natural tendencies in an environment we were never really suited for, just like a polar bear stuck in the desert.

The moral of the polar bear story is that your weight problem is far from being totally your fault. Just know that a certain number of factors that are simply out of your control have brought you to the point where you are today. On the other hand, this does not mean there is nothing you can do about your weight. Indeed, there are many things you can do to get a good handle on the situation. That's what this book is all about.

Know, too, that it's probably not going to be as bad as you might think. The research clearly shows us that if you lose just 5–10 percent of what you weigh today, this can lead to a substantial decrease in your risk of developing heart disease and diabetes (NIH, 1998). And believe me, it is possible. I know this to be true because other ordinary people just like you have done it in controlled studies, *when they used the right strategies*.

Chapter 1 in a Nutshell

- ◆ The medical name for fat is adipose tissue.

- ◆ Fat cells called adipocytes make up adipose tissue.

- ◆ Adipocytes can greatly expand to hold much fat.

- ◆ When they get bigger, you get bigger.

- ◆ Your body puts fat in the adipocyte when you eat more food than your body needs at the moment. It's storing energy for the future.

- ◆ Your body takes fat out of the adipocyte when you have given it a smaller supply of energy to run on than it needs (a diet strategy) or when you burn up more energy than you've given it that day (an exercise strategy). When adipocytes get smaller, you get smaller and weigh less.

◆ Cellulite is caused by irregular patterns of connective tissue right under the skin.

◆ The fat in cellulite is no different from any other kind of fat.

◆ Spot reducing is not possible.

◆ Calculating your BMI is a great way to classify your weight level and know where you stand.

◆ A BMI of 25 or above puts you at risk for many health problems.

◆ People with a tendency to put on extra fat in the stomach area are at increased risk for health problems than those who carry extra fat on their hips and/or thighs.

◆ Measuring your waist circumference is a good way to assess your abdominal fat content.

◆ Men with a waist circumference of more than 40 inches and women with a waist circumference of more than 35 inches are at increased risk for health problems.

◆ There may be factors, such as the natural tendency to overeat, that contribute to your weight problem and that are out of your control. Focus your energy on the ones that are in your control.

2

How to Get Yourself Motivated

The best plan in the world is useless if it's never carried out.

This is an action book. I wrote it with ten fingers, a keyboard, and a stack of research articles never more than a foot away. The diet and exercise strategies that I describe in simple language in the pages that follow were published in respected medical journals and have been proven effective through rigorous clinical trials. After reading such a practical book of proven strategies, I ask you, who could possibly fail in their attempt to lose weight? A lot of people could, if all this book had to offer was a plan.

I have been educating patients in changing their health habits for a long time now, and it is my opinion that there are at least two essential ingredients everyone needs to reach *any* goal. First you need the "tools" that give you a possible way of getting to your goal. Then, you need *motivation*—that is, the desire to pick up those tools and put them to use. If you stop and think about it for a minute, having just one of these two things is simply not enough, as one without the other will get you nowhere fast. On the other hand, having both propels you to your target.

With this thinking, I designed this book to meet the needs of both the person who lacks tools and the person who lacks motivation. This shouldn't leave anyone out, because if you had both, you probably wouldn't be reading this book.

The tools you need to lose weight—that is, the diet and exercise strategies—are covered in the remainder of this book. What you are reading at the moment, however, will prompt a little soul-searching that will hopefully give you the necessary fuel to put the diet and exercise strategies to good use.

THE FORMULA THAT WORKS WONDERS

The famous martial arts expert Bruce Lee was once quoted as saying, "Knowing is not enough, we must apply." Will Rogers said it a bit differently, "Even if you're on the right track you'll get run over if you just sit there." There is much wisdom in these statements. One can know exactly how to accomplish a goal to the very last detail, but without the motivation to carry it out and execute it, one will never succeed.

I see this literally every single day, without fail, in the hospital where I work. Patients know they need to exercise regularly, watch their diet, control their blood sugar, or even take their prescribed medications. The overwhelming majority of these people also have a good idea how to accomplish these kinds of goals. The problem is, *they lack the motivation to do so*.

So what is the answer for those who fit into this category? My answer is simply this: When confronted with a task that you lack the motivation to do, find a reason to do it that gives you something you really want. In other words, *what's in it for you?*

Sound a bit too simplistic? Let me illustrate my point using exercise as an example. Everybody knows they should exercise more because it's the healthy thing to do. Still, this reason for exercising, however strongly supported by research and logical it is, usually fails to motivate the majority of people to immediately put on their sneakers and, say, start walking a little bit every day. Why? Because the reason just isn't a powerful enough motivator on its own. Sure, being healthy is a good thing, we all know this, but it just doesn't always give people enough juice to get going, perhaps because it's not specific enough.

Now let's look at the same goal, getting yourself to start walking for exercise, from a slightly different angle. What if I told you that walking every day would help get that extra fat off your stomach or thighs? Now this is a little more appealing and more specific than walking just to "be healthier." Let's keep going. What if I told you that walking would help you get that extra fat off your stomach or thighs *and* you'd start getting more looks and attention from members of the opposite sex? Sounding better all the time? How about if I told you that walking might even have positive effects on your sex life? I bet *that* would motivate more people to start walking than just telling them to start exercising because "it's healthy."

I once gave a home exercise to a patient who was a real nonexercise kind of gal. Even though it was a very simple exercise for strengthening her back muscles, I still felt that my chances were slim to none that she would actually go home and do it. Knowing that she just *hated* exercise, I also slipped in the fact that not only would this exercise strengthen her back muscles, but it would also tone up her hips and thighs as well. What woman wouldn't want that? Do you think she ended up doing the exercise faithfully?

Along the same lines, I tried for years to get my wife to lift weights. An avid weight lifter myself, I could see and feel the benefits every day and always encouraged her to start strength training whenever we went to the gym. Oh, I would pull out all of my physical therapy facts to encourage her. I would say things like, "Just think, honey, you would hardly have to watch what you eat if you lifted weights. Building muscle increases your metabolism, making your body burn more calories." Or there was the old scare 'em tactic: "Did you know that as we get older we start to lose muscle mass?"

Of course she knew that strength training was good for her and all that stuff. Unfortunately, all these discussions ever amounted to was her trying it a time or two and sticking with it for no more than a few weeks at a time. I eventually dropped the whole issue, as it was clear that weight lifting just wasn't her cup of tea. In fact, she downright hated it. Then one day, years later, something strange happened. Out of the clear blue sky she asked me if I would help her to begin a weight lifting routine at the YMCA. Although somewhat shocked, I didn't question her and quickly agreed.

A day or so later, my wife and I were eating dinner, and she began telling me about a coworker (who happened to be around the same age) who had recently been screened for osteoporosis and was found to have a slight decrease in her bone mass. While this wasn't a major problem, it still was rather unexpected for someone her coworker's age. Not surprisingly, the doctor recommended a treatment that is proven to increase bone density: strength training.

Now it all made sense. Not wanting to end up with the brittle bones her friend was headed for, my wife had latched onto this new, motivating reason to exercise that would give her something she really wanted: stronger bones and no osteoporosis. Interestingly enough, no other reason that I had brought to her attention in the past, however sound and logical, scary or research-based, was ever quite enough to get her to hit the weights.

To this day, she continues to lift weights every week, despite her total lack of love for this particular activity.

A similar change occurred in two nurses I once worked with in a large teaching hospital. They had smoked daily for years until one month it happened that they both became pregnant. It was at this time that they made the decision to quit smoking, *and succeeded.*

Yes, these two nurses, surely addicted to nicotine by this time, managed to kick the habit shortly thereafter. The reason? It was because the payout behind it all had changed. They were pregnant and knew smoking was a health hazard to their babies, so they stopped—just like that. No if, ands, or butts (pardon the pun). Where the motivating reason they had before to quit smoking (bad for your health) was not powerful enough, the new motivating factor (harmful to a baby's health) did the trick. Stop and think about this for a minute. The desired behavior, to quit smoking, never changed a bit, *only the motivating factor behind it did.*

By changing just the thinking and reasoning behind this most difficult task, they managed to make a seemingly impossible change. Remember, *if you have trouble getting yourself to do something, find a reason to do it that gives you something you really want.*

I often explain these concepts to my physical-therapy students when discussing how to motivate difficult patients who refuse to participate in their physical therapy. One common scenario involves stair climbing. Before a patient goes home from a hospital stay, physical therapists usually like to make sure that the patient can climb stairs, particularly if he or she will have to do so in order to get into the house. Most patients, having been sick for quite some time, and far from being in the best shape of their life, are understandably quite hesitant to tackle stairs. Some patients do it and get it over with, a few put up a fuss and then do it, and some others refuse altogether.

A first-year student I was teaching one day wondered what happened to those patients who refused to try climbing stairs. "I mean, after all," the student said, "some of them have to climb many stairs just to get into their house. What will they do if they get to their front door and can't make it in?"

I explained to the student that at this point the motivation factor of these patients for climbing stairs has totally changed. "When we ask patients to climb stairs here in the hospital," I said, "most patients are climbing them only because we are making them do so. The stairs aren't really taking them anywhere. When they get home, though, and stand in front of their house, the motivation to climb the stairs they see before them is their home, their own bed, and their loved ones who lie beyond the steps."

Once again, you can see from this example that the task hasn't changed one iota. Steps are steps, whether they're in a hospital or at a house. However, once the reason behind climbing the stairs has changed—giving the patient something they *really* want—the motivation to do the task is no longer a problem at all, no matter how hard the task may seem.

Want the *Cliffs Notes* version? Action springs from desire. And if you really start thinking about it, you'll soon see that this principle is already well at work every day. The table on page 25 gives a few examples of how people do things that they don't like to do all the time, just by having a powerful motivating factor:

Let's pull all of this together now and put it to practical use. You have in your hands a book of diet and exercise strategies that have been proven by research to help you lose weight. From here, one of the following two scenarios is likely:

♦ If you are a real self starter and feel like you've got plenty of motivation to carry out the strategies that follow, then you will more than likely succeed in shedding pounds and improving your health.

♦ On the other hand, maybe the desire is there, but you find you just don't have quite enough oomph to start carrying out the strategies. This means you haven't found a truly meaningful motivating factor yet. Therefore, the next step is to *find a reason to begin that gives you something you really want.*

So what do you want? Losing weight could mean

♦ not ending up like someone you know who is in poor health

♦ setting a good example for your kids to follow

Old behavior	Motivating factor	What the motivating factor can give you that you want	New behavior
can't quit smoking	just diagnosed with lung cancer	longer life	you quit smoking
not much for reading books	your best friend just wrote a book —you're in it	find out what they said about you	you read a book
always late to work	your boss said if you're late again, you're fired	keep your job	you're on time
can't stand country music	someone hot has tickets to a concert and asks you out	a hot date	you go to the concert and listen to country music
hate sitting in traffic	have to get to job to earn a living	money and health-insurance benefits	you sit in traffic
hate a bad-tasting medicine	want to be healthy	feel well again	take the bad-tasting medicine
hate long car rides	see family	an enjoyable visit with your family	go on a long car ride
don't eat right; don't get enough exercise	?	?	control eating; exercise more

- ◆ better sex
- ◆ more energy
- ◆ living longer, giving you added years to spend with your loved ones
- ◆ making an existing health problem less severe
- ◆ just feeling better
- ◆ more confidence
- ◆ getting into shape to do things you have never done before
- ◆ looking better
- ◆ feeling strong and fit again
- ◆ decreasing your chances of having to get a joint replacement
- ◆ your clothes fitting better

Just a few suggestions to think about. Remember, above all else, *in order for the motivating factor to work it must be meaningful and give you something you really want.* Unfortunately, I can only help you by offering some suggestions. From there, the ball is entirely in your court, because nobody else in the world knows *your* best motivating factor but you. But believe me, it most certainly exists. The time is now, today, this very minute, and you're up to bat. What will your motivating factor be? Go back to the table on page 25: What is going to get you from the old behavior on the left side of the table to the new behavior on the right? Look at the last entry in the table: Can you fill in the boxes that contain question marks *and change your life?*

Of course you can. As you will see later (in the chapter on successful dieters), others have managed to find a motivating factor that allows them to effectively carry out a weight-loss plan over the long run. And if others have, *then so can you.* Then, once you have discovered your motivating factor, you definitely will have won at least half the battle. The door will finally unlock and you'll be well on your way to reaching your weight-loss goals. You will have gained the ability to apply the knowledge that you are about to learn in the pages that lie ahead.

Chapter 2 in a Nutshell

◆ The best plan in the world, no matter how good, is totally useless until it is put into action.

◆ Action springs from motivation.

◆ Rest assured that you can accomplish just about anything if you can find the right motivating factor.

◆ A motivating factor must be meaningful and must give you something you really want.

3

Surefire Ways to *Fail* at Losing Weight

Knowing the past can prevent future mistakes and make your path clearer.

You're problably thinking: What's this? A chapter on how to *fail* at losing weight? Funny, I thought this book was about how to *succeed* at losing weight.

Before you think I've gone bonkers, I'd better explain.

You're at a place now where you're ready to forge ahead. You are able to move forward with confidence because you have found your motivating factor, which allows you to push through barriers that have held you back in the past. And you discovered this motivation because you have dug down deep, perhaps deeper than most people ever do.

But before beginning your quest for a healthier body, I think it's a good idea to first take a brief look at the research on various diet and exercise treatments that have been used to lose weight. Why? To take advantage of the past and see what really has and has not worked. Dispelling weight-loss folklore once and for all can keep you from wasting future time and energy and, quite possibly for the first time ever, allow you to focus entirely on strategies that have been proven in scientific studies to actually help. In other words, today the buck stops here!

So with all these thoughts in mind, I've meticulously searched through the medical library for you and have put literally decades of weight-loss research *right in your very hands.* If you have a magnifying glass, dust it off because we're going to be taking a close look at some rather eye-opening studies!

THE TRUTH ABOUT DIETING AS A WEIGHT-LOSS STRATEGY

Anyone who jumps into the research on diets will quickly notice one thing: *There's a million of 'em!*

Although the sheer number of diets that humans have concocted over the years will make even the most hard-core researcher's head spin, I have found that there are *two* main characteristics that seem to set apart the various weight-loss diets. They are

- a diet's calorie content, which is how many total calories it lets you eat per day, and

- a diet's composition, which is the amount of fat vs. protein vs. carbohydrate it allows.

Of these two characteristics, we really only need to be concerned with a diet's calorie content when evaluating its ability to cause weight loss. As you will find out later in this chapter, a particular diet's ability to make you shed fat depends more on *the number of calories it provides* than it does on *the types of foods that give you those calories.*

Once you have an idea of how many calories a diet lets

you have each day, you will then likely be able to put it into one of these three main diet categories:

- ◆ fasting, which gives you zero calories a day

- ◆ a very low calorie diet, which gives you between 250 and 800 calories a day

- ◆ a low-calorie diet, which gives you between 800 and 1,500 calories a day

Where did I get these categories from? From the research. If you dig up studies that have tested weight-loss diets and lay them all out on a table, you'll soon find that most of them can be roughly sorted out into one of the above three categories. Grouping diets like this is an easy and convenient way of looking at the diet research for some answers, because these three diet categories not only include most of the diets that exist, but they also consist of the most thoroughly researched ones.

From now on, whenever you hear or read about the latest and greatest diet plan, I want you to get into the habit of asking yourself one question: How many calories does it provide? That's how scientists in studies often size up diet plans that they are going to test, and that's precisely the way we're going to be looking at them in this book. Then, once you know what category a particular diet belongs to, you can use the information from this chapter to tell you which ones *really* work and which ones are clearly a hit-or-miss venture.

A Diet's Calorie Content

Let's take a closer look at each of the three main diet categories.

Total Fasting

If eating too much makes you fat, then all you have to do to get skinny is *stop* eating, right?

You're probably grinning a bit at the moment, but believe it or not, this strategy to lose weight was actually used at one time. To be precise, it was called "total fasting." I prefer to call it what it really is: *starvation*.

Yep, believe it or not, at one time total fasting was well on its way to becoming a bona fide medical treatment for the severely overweight. It was around the 1950s and 60s in particular that studies on fasting began cropping up with noticeable frequency, showing that it was indeed possible for a person to lose remarkable amounts of weight by eating not so much as a morsel of food. In a typical fasting scenario, a person would be forbidden to eat any carbohydrates, proteins, or fats over a prolonged stretch of time, but would be allowed plenty of water to drink. Strangely, and contrary to what you'd expect, it has been well documented that many individuals actually lose the hunger sensation after the first few days of no eating.

A good example of the fasting research going on around that time is a 1959 study conducted at Piedmont Hospital in Atlanta, Georgia, which reported that its nine patients lost an average of 19 *pounds* after just one week of total fasting!

Not too shabby, huh? Of course the research continued, and like a lot of things, people began to think that if some fasting is good, then more *must* be better. In 1973, the peer-reviewed *Postgraduate Medical Journal* published a case report of a twenty-seven-year-old man who, under medical supervision, had successfully fasted for an amazing duration of 382 days!

The patient, weighing in initially at 456 pounds, lost an astounding 276 pounds over the course of this marathon fast, eventually tipping the scales at 180 when all was said and done. Not surprising, though, is the fact that this individual also made it into the *Guinness Book of Records!*

Unfortunately, what seemed to be a surefire way of getting people to lose unhealthy amounts of weight was soon met with the ultimate side effect—death. Many people lost massive amounts of weight on total fasts, but the literature also began to report an alarming number of people dying after prolonged periods of fasting. As a result, and since long-term studies showed that many patients ended up regaining their lost pounds, enthusiasm quickly faded, and total fasting as a weight-loss treatment was basically put out to pasture.

Very Low Calorie Diets
Spurred by the remarkable weight losses that took place in people who fasted, it seemed as if a search began to find the lowest-calorie diet possible that could avoid the dangers of total starvation but still produce dramatic weight loss.

When researchers looked back at experiences with fasting, it was noted that while people did lose a lot of fat, they also lost large amounts of protein. Because of this phenomenon, diets loaded with protein were soon developed and thus popularized what is known as the *very low calorie diet*. Given commonly in liquid form, these diets typically provided the dieter with around 250 to 800 calories a day.

This was around the 1970s and 80s, and it seemed that just about everyone was jumping on the very-low-calorie-diet bandwagon. Here are a few popular ones you may have heard of:

- the "last-chance" diet
- Optifast
- Modifast
- the Cambridge diet

With their low calorie content, there was no question that these diets could indeed cause rapid weight loss. Unfortunately, reports of heart problems and sudden death with the use of liquid protein diets led to investigations of their use. Fifty-eight deaths were reported in 1977 and 1978, which caused both the Food and Drug Administration (FDA) and Centers for Disease Control (CDC) to terminate the use of very low calorie diets until further studies could assure their safety. Interestingly, the low quantity and poor quality of the protein, as well as their prolonged use without proper medical supervision, have been cited as reasons for these deaths.

After such awful events as these, one would expect that the story of the very low calorie diet would be over in a hurry. Surprisingly, very low calorie diets did *not* fall out of favor like total fasting had, and they actually continued to be modified over the years. Higher-quality protein was added, as well as carbohydrates, fats, vitamins, and essential minerals. There has also been a noticeable rise in the number of calories provided in these diets, with the total calorie intake going from approximately 360 to 600 calories a day originally, to about 420 to 800 calories in later products.

So the million-dollar question now is, where are we *today* with very low calorie diets? Are they safe? Are they effective?

To get to the bottom of these questions, we once again turn to the scientific literature for some answers. First of all, are they safe? Yes, with some qualifications. According to an extensive review published in *The Journal of the American Medical Association* in 1993, it was concluded that "current very low calorie diets are generally safe when used under proper medical supervision in moderately and severely obese patients."

Okay, so it seems that their safety has been vastly improved. Next, are they effective?

In medicine, the only way to really answer this question with certainty is to conduct what is called a *randomized controlled trial*. This is a kind of study where you take a group of people and randomly divide them into two (or more) groups. One group gets to try a test diet that you think might be the most effective—let's say, the tree-bark diet—while another becomes a *control group*, whose members stay on their regular diets for comparison. Next you let the test-diet group try out the tree-bark diet for a period of time, say six weeks, at the same time as the control-group members stay on their regular diets.

If at the end of the six weeks the tree-bark-diet group lost significantly more weight than the control group did on a regular diet, one can then really say that the tree-bark diet is indeed effective and better than a regular diet. On the other hand, if the tree-bark-diet group lost just as much weight as the control group did on a regular diet, it can be said that both diets are equally effective for losing weight. Pretty nifty setup, huh?

As you might have guessed, the *real* power of the randomized controlled trial lies in the fact that it has a comparison, or control, group. It's this control group that gives researchers something to compare results to, which allows them to figure out just how effective a new diet really is. If you stop and think about it for a minute, how else would you *really* know how good a new diet is unless you formally compare it to something else?

As far as I'm concerned, *nobody* had darn well better say that they have a diet that is effective *unless* they have a randomized controlled trial to back up what they say. The randomized controlled trial is the highest proof in medicine that a diet (or any other treatment, for that matter) is effective. Drugs, for example, are tested in randomized controlled trials all the time. I don't think anyone reading this book would want to try the latest pain pill, surgical procedure, or chemotherapy treatment unless it had *really* been proven to be effective and helpful. Why then, I ask, shouldn't we apply this exact same logic to diets as well?

Now that you know the right way to determine if a diet is actually proven to be effective, let's go back to the question "Are very low calorie diets effective?"

In the short run, yes, they are faster than a speeding locomotive. However, over the long haul, randomized controlled trials tell us that they actually do *no better* than higher-calorie diets! A prime example is a 1994 study published in *The Journal of Consulting and Clinical Psychology* that took forty-nine obese women and randomly placed them into one of two groups:

◆ those who were put on a 1,200-calorie diet for a year

or

◆ those who were put on a 420-calorie (i.e., very low calorie) diet for four months, followed by a 1,200-calorie diet for the rest of the year

Both groups also received behavioral therapy (to help them get social support, slow the rate of eating, and so on) and were started on an exercise program (mainly walking) two months into the study. Additionally, each group participated in a six-month weight-maintenance program at the end of the year of dieting. Therefore, what we now have are two groups, equal in all things, *except* the calorie intake of their diets.

And the results? As one would expect, the people on the 420-calorie diet for four months lost far more weight than those who followed a 1,200-calorie diet during that same time period. As a matter of fact, they actually lost *twice as much weight*.

However, although it seemed like the very low calorie diet was going to be the clear winner, the long-term results surprisingly told another story. Follow-up one and a half years later showed that each person in the 420-calorie group had lost, on average, a grand total of 24 pounds, while each person in the 1,200-calorie group lost 27 pounds—not enough of a difference between the two to write home about. Other studies comparing very low calorie diets to low-calorie diets in both the short and long run have also reached similar conclusions (Wadden, 1989; Wadden, 1990; Wing, 1994).

It appears, then, that the bottom line for the person trying to lose weight is that that there really is no long-term advantage of *very low* calorie diets over *low*-calorie diets. In fact, following either type will eventually land you at the same place, so why bother losing weight on a skimpy 420-calorie diet when you will do just as well on a more plentiful 1,200-calorie one?

At this point, some readers may be thinking, "Why not just *stay* on the very low calorie diet to lose weight?" Basically, the answer to this is because very low calorie diets are used as a *temporary* means of reducing excessive weight. Like fasting, it's not the kind of thing you can keep doing for the rest of your life. Furthermore, there is little published data on the safety of the exclusive use of very low calorie diets for longer than four months.

So there you have it, the real deal about very low calorie diets, according to randomized controlled trials. They are safe (when done under medical supervision) and do indeed cause drastic amounts of weight loss. Over time, though, they provide the same results as *low*-calorie diets. Which brings us to...

Low-Calorie Diets

The medical literature says that a low-calorie diet is one that gives you somewhere between 800 and 1,500 calories a day.

This is the diet strategy I recommend in this book for the average person trying to lose weight. As usual, I have several good reasons for this choice, *all based upon randomized controlled trials*. They are the following:

◆ It is *proven* that low-calorie diets cause people to lose weight (Katzel, 1995).

◆ When people are placed on low-calorie diets and are followed for a period of years, studies have shown that they *consistently* lose more weight than people in the control group (Stamler, 1987).

◆ Studies show that low-calorie diets cause people to lose abdominal fat, a risk factor for conditions such as heart disease and stroke (Dengel, 1995).

◆ As previously discussed, low-calorie diets cause people to lose just as much weight in the long term as diets with fewer calories (Wadden, 1994).

Now that you have more facts right at your fingertips, picking the best diet for losing weight should be much easier to do. For the average person looking to reduce their weight, you can see that a low-calorie diet is hard to beat.

A Diet's Composition

Up to now we have looked at the ideal diet for losing weight in terms of how many calories the diet contains. The other thing to think about is the diet's composition (what it's made up of)—or more simply put, what percentage of carbohydrates, fats, and proteins should make up those calories? For instance, is a 1,000-calorie, *high*-carbohydrate diet better than a 1,000-calorie, *low*-carbohydrate diet? (And while we're talking about carbohydrates, which is better, simple or complex carbs?) Or can you lose more weight on a 1,000-calorie, *high-fat* diet instead?

Welcome to what is probably the most hotly debated topic concerning weight-loss diets. While you can find a lot of people quickly taking a side on this issue and pointing out miscellaneous medical facts or talking about how their Uncle Joe lost 50 pounds eating bacon and eggs every day, it is best to settle the issue by once again taking a good look at well-conducted medical studies published in peer-reviewed journals. Let's have a peek and see what some of the research has to say about all of this:

◆ *The Journal of the American Dietetic Association*
published the results of a study where thirty-five
overweight females were all put on a 1,200-calorie-
a-day diet and then divided into three groups (Alford, 1990). One group followed a diet containing
75 percent carbohydrates, another group 45 percent
carbohydrates, and the last group 25 percent carbohydrates. Variations in fat and protein made up the
rest of the diet patterns. After ten weeks, each
1,200-calorie diet had contributed to weight loss,
*but there were no significant differences in weight loss
among the groups.*

◆ *The International Journal of Obesity* published a
study that took twenty-five obese individuals and
put them all on an 800-calorie-a-day diet (Piatti,
1993). This time, the carbohydrates were further
broken down into the simple and complex kind.
Subjects were put into one of three groups: group
one (whose diet was made up of 45 percent complex
carbohydrates, 15 percent simple carbohydrates, 20
percent fat, and 20 percent protein), group two (15
percent complex carbohydrates, 45 percent simple
carbohydrates, 20 percent fat, 20 percent protein),
and group three (15 percent complex carbohydrates,
5 percent simple carbohydrates, 60 percent fat, 20
percent protein). The results? *A similar decrease in
body weight was observed in all three groups.*

◆ *The American Journal of Clinical Nutrition* published a study that took forty-three obese patients
and randomly put them on one of two diets (Golay,
1996). Each diet contained a total of 1,000 calories a

day, but one diet was made up of 53 percent fat, 15 percent carbohydrates, 32 percent protein, while the other consisted of 26 percent fat, 45 percent carbohydrates, 29 percent protein. *At the end of the six-week study period, there were no significant differences in the amount of weight lost between the two groups.*

As you can see, despite numerous studies feeding overweight individuals a great many different combinations of carbohydrates, fats, and proteins, *everyone loses similar amounts of weight as long as they are all eating the same number of calories.*

Now that's some practical information you can quickly put to use when looking at weight-loss diets. Don't be fooled into thinking that that there is some undiscovered, "magic" combination of foods out there that will instantly melt the fat away. Clearly, the published research is pointing in just one direction: *It's the total amount of calories you eat every day that really determines if you will lose weight, not a certain proportion of carbohydrates, fats, or protein.*

There will, of course, be many books, television commercials, and magazine articles that would have you believe otherwise. Just as exercise fads come and go, so do diets, all proclaiming to offer the best combination of foods to make the pounds miraculously fly off.

Perhaps the latest winner of this ongoing popularity contest has been the low-carbohydrate diet. Those who promote this type of diet say that carbohydrates are the enemy and that protein and fats should make up most of our diet each day. "Eat that cheeseburger (without the bun) and watch those carbs," they say, "and the weight will surely come off." It's quite catchy and is probably every dieter's dream come true. Once again, however, the research sets things straight.

A study published in the prestigious *New England Journal of Medicine* put to test what is perhaps the king of all low-carbohydrate diets—the Atkins diet (Foster, 2003). Sixty-three obese men and women were randomly assigned to either a low-carbohydrate, high-fat Atkins diet or to a regular low-calorie diet (high carbohydrate, low fat). At this point, the following results of this long-term randomized controlled trial shouldn't surprise you one bit:

◆ After six months, the group that was given a copy of *Dr. Atkins' New Diet Revolution* and instructed to read it and follow the diet as described lost more weight than the group that followed a regular low-calorie diet.

◆ After one year, however, *there were no significant differences in weight loss between the two groups.*

I don't know about you, but I'm thinking that some diets really aren't that revolutionary when properly tested in an unbiased, randomized controlled trial. This study in particular was very well done because it carried out its observations over a full year so it could really determine how long the results would last. While at six months it looked like the low-carbohydrate diet was the best thing since sliced bread, a careful follow-up proved otherwise.

Once again, people who consumed a high-fat diet did no better in the long run than those who ate a regular low-fat diet, making this study yet another example of the fact that it matters very little (in terms of weight loss) how you shuffle around your fats, carbohydrates, or proteins. As piles of studies repeatedly point out, the bottom line always comes down to calories, calories, calories.

THE TRUTH ABOUT EXERCISE AS A WEIGHT-LOSS STRATEGY

Let's say you and a friend would both like to lose some weight. You and she plan to try walking a little after dinner each day in order to burn some calories. However, your friend says she is just too busy right now and will catch up with you next month. Four weeks go by. Who would you guess is most likely to have lost some weight, you or your friend?

Although the answer might seem obvious, the truth is that it really depends on whether you're a man or a woman. The overweight woman who walks for one hour a day, without dieting, will in all likelihood lose *no weight* over a month's time. On the other hand, an overweight man walking for an hour each day would. Surprised? Let me explain.

I once conducted a literature search to find out exactly what the research had to say about exercising to lose weight. I specifically looked for randomized controlled trials, because as you now know, these are the best proof in medicine that a treatment really works. Shortly after beginning what I thought was going to be a cut-and-dried review, I came across the following study:

The Archives of Internal Medicine published a study that took 131 overweight men and women and randomized them into either an exercise group or a control group

(Donnelly, 2003). No changes in diet were made in either group. The exercise group underwent sixteen months of supervised exercise, mainly walking on a treadmill, working up to forty-five minutes per session. The control group continued with life as usual. At the end of the sixteen months, men who exercised showed significant *decreases* in body weight compared to the control group, while women who exercised *maintained* their weight.

Shocked at the fact that a group of overweight women could actually do verified exercise five days a week for well over a year and still fail to drop a single pound, I began to dig further and further into the research to see if this study was just a fluke or if exercise really was a poor way for women to lose weight.

Many journal articles later, when all was said and done, two trends in the literature became quite obvious. The first was that for overweight or obese men, the majority of randomized controlled trials clearly proved that exercise alone (in other words, without dieting) *could* result in weight loss. Here are some typical examples of what I found:

- ◆ A randomized controlled trial published in *The American Journal of Cardiology* showed that forty-two overweight men who exercised under supervision for one hour, three days a week (as well as being instructed to increase their routine activity), lost weight compared to the control group. Exercise consisted of calisthenics, walking, jogging, or running (Fortmann, 1988).

- ◆ A one-year randomized controlled trial published in *The New England Journal of Medicine* showed that overweight men who engaged in walking or jogging (eventually working up to forty to fifty minutes per session) had significant loss of total body weight compared to the control group (Wood, 1988).

The second trend in the research concerned females. Astonishingly, the majority of randomized controlled trials I could find that had taken a group of overweight or obese women and put them on an exercise program (again, without changing their diet) showed *no significant weight loss whatsoever* (Donnelly, 2003; Nieman, 2002; Utter, 2000; Hinkleman, 1993; King, 1991; Hagan, 1986). Here are a few examples:

◆ *The Journal of Sports Medicine and Physical Fitness* published a study that took fifty overweight women and randomized them into either an exercise group or a control group (Hinkleman, 1993). After fifteen weeks of walking for forty-five minutes a day, five days a week, no weight loss occurred in the exercise group.

◆ A randomized controlled trial published in *The Journal of the American College of Nutrition* studied obese females who walked for forty-five minutes, five days a week (Nieman, 2002). After twelve weeks of exercising, there were no significant changes in body mass in the exercise group compared to the control group.

For some reason, perhaps because men have more muscle and thus burn more calories during a given activity than women, *exercising alone to lose weight does not affect everyone the same way*. This may be a most unpopular conclusion, especially coming from a physical therapist, but if one is willing to dig up the studies, lay them all out on a table, and scrutinize their results as I have done, the facts are the facts.

Now, does this mean that this book does *not* recommend exercise as a strategy to lose weight? Absolutely not. As you will see shortly, exercise must be done *in combination* with other strategies in order for it to be a truly effective part of a weight-loss plan for both men and women. To further illustrate, let's use you and your fictitious friend once again.

Pretend now that you are still walking a little each day after dinner in your effort to lose weight, while your friend, still much too busy to exercise, decides to go on a diet instead. Another month passes. *Now* who will lose more weight over a four-week period?

If you said that your friend would win the race to Skinnyville, congratulations, you're right on the money! The research distinctly shows diet strategies beating out exercise strategies when one is trying to lose weight, and this applies *equally* to men and women. Here's one such example:

◆ A randomized controlled trial published in *The American Journal of Cardiology* compared dieting men and women to exercising men and women. After three months, dieters lost more weight than those who exercised (Gordon, 1997).

Looks like dieting is the way to go then when it comes to losing weight, right? Not so fast. Let's have a look at one last scenario.

Imagine that by this time you're becoming *extremely* disappointed, because you can't help but notice that your busy friend is losing way more weight than you just by dieting. A little frustrated, you decide it's time to shake things up a bit. It's time for a plan B.

Since you do find walking quite relaxing at the end of the day, even though you haven't lost any weight yet, you choose to keep it up. But since walking hasn't gotten you exactly where you want to be in terms of losing weight, you decide to also start a diet, just like your friend did. At this point you are dieting *and* exercising, while your busy friend continues to just diet. Four more weeks fly by. Now who is winning the battle of the bulge?

Congratulations, this time *you're* in the driver's seat! Your new plan of combining dieting and exercising is a complete and utter success. Rooting for you also are piles of research clearly showing the superiority of using both diet *and* exercise strategies together when trying to lose weight, such as the following:

- A study published in *Medicine and Science in Sports and Exercise* took forty-eight men and forty-eight women, all overweight, and randomly assigned them to one of four groups: diet and exercise, diet only, exercise only, and a control group (Hagan, 1986). Men and women who both dieted and exercised lost significantly more body weight than those who only dieted or only exercised.

- A study published in the *International Journal of Obesity* analyzed twenty-five years worth of weight-loss research to determine the effectiveness of dieting, exercising, or dieting plus exercising. It was concluded that in the long term, diet plus exercise was superior to just dieting or just exercising (Miller, 1997).

Which strategy causes you to lose more weight?	
	... and the winner is:
dieting *or* doing nothing	dieting
exercising *or* doing nothing	exercise if you're a man; neither one if you're woman
exercising *or* dieting	dieting
dieting + exercising *or* dieting	dieting + exercising
dieting + exercising *or* exercising	dieting + exercising

Okay. We've covered a lot of ground so far about how diet and exercise stack up as weight-loss strategies. Now let's see how we can put all this research together so you can put it to practical use *today*. The table above, based strictly on randomized controlled trials that have rigorously tested diet and exercise strategies to lose weight, shows that exercise by itself (when done in practical amounts) is not really that effective unless it is combined with some sort of a diet strategy.

If more people knew this information, I'd be willing to bet that a lot of time and effort could be saved trying to lose weight. Most readers can probably name someone who suddenly started walking a little each day or decided to join a gym to lose weight, only to quit after a matter of weeks because the meager payout just wasn't worth all the hard work. As you can see, sometimes a little knowledge can make the difference between spinning your wheels or actually getting the results you're after.

Here's the moral of the story: If you want a surefire way to fail at losing weight, just ignore the medically proven knowledge about weight-loss strategies.

ENTER THE DIANEX STRATEGY

As you have just learned from reading this chapter, the real power of diet and exercise comes when they are *combined*. It is with this thinking that I have coined the term *Dianex Strategy*, which is what you get when you put a <u>di</u>et <u>an</u>d <u>ex</u>ercise strategy together.

Fueled by your motivating factor, the Dianex Strategy is based purely on scientific research and offers a truly no-nonsense approach to weight loss—thus providing you with the proper tools to reach your weight-loss goals once and for all!

Chapter 3 in a Nutshell

◆ The only way to be sure that a diet is really effective or "works" is by properly testing it in a controlled trial or, better yet, in a randomized controlled trial. The randomized controlled trial is the highest form of proof in medicine that a treatment is really effective.

◆ *Fasting,* which provides the dieter with zero calories, can cause one to lose much weight in a short period of time. It does, however, have poor long-term results and has even been known to cause death.

◆ *Very low calorie diets,* which provide between 250 and 800 calories a day, can cause one to lose much weight but in the long run are no more effective than

low-calorie diets, according to randomized controlled trials.

◆ *Low-calorie diets,* which provide between 800 and
1,500 calories a day, have been proven to work in
randomized controlled trials, cause people to lose
abdominal fat, and are just as effective as diets that
provide fewer calories, making them the best choice
for weight loss.

◆ Numerous studies have proven that it is the total
number of calories you eat every day that determines if you will lose weight, not a certain proportion
of carbohydrates, fats, or protein.

◆ A combination of exercising and dieting will cause
you to lose more weight than either dieting or exercising alone.

4

The Diet Strategy

Once you've got good eating habits, they're just as
hard to break as the bad ones.

*E*very weight-loss diet I know of seems to have one
thing in common. Do know what it is? Okay, I'll give
you a hint. Take a look at some of these popular diet plans
and give me your best guess:

- ◆ Weight Watchers—limits calories by limiting points

- ◆ Protein Power—limits calories by limiting sweets
  and starchy carbohydrates

- ◆ The Zone—limits calories by limiting blocks

- ◆ Atkins Diet—limits calories by limiting carbohydrates

- ◆ Body for Life—limits calories by limiting both portion size and number of portions

- ◆ Slim Fast—limits calories using special shakes

- ◆ Food Guide Pyramid—limits calories by limiting
  servings

- ◆ 8 Minutes in the Morning—limits calorie intake

- ◆ Nutrisystem—limits calories by controlling portions

◆ South Beach Diet—limits calories by limiting portion size and carbohydrates

◆ Sugar Busters—limits calories by limiting portion size and refined sugar

◆ Jenny Craig—limits calorie intake

Have you figured out yet what they all have in common? Alright, maybe my hint was a little *too* big.

If you guessed that every weight-loss diet *limits calories* one way or another, you're absolutely right. Some limit a person's total calorie intake outright (e.g., by putting you on a 1,200-calorie-a-day diet), while others simply restrict the kinds of foods you can eat (e.g., the Atkins diet limits carbohydrates such as soft drinks and sweets made with real sugars, which helps lower overall calorie intake). Any way you slice it, it's an inescapable fact that they all limit calories. Isn't it interesting how weight-loss diets all start to look the same once they've been stripped of colorful promises, testimonials, and flashy before-and-after pictures?

You betcha. *The unavoidable truth is that* all *successful weight-loss diets work for the exact same reason: They give your body a smaller supply of calories (energy) to run on, which forces you to use up your fat stores.* Period. No ifs, ands, or buts. Show me a weight-loss diet that works and I'll show you a diet that in one way or another restricts calorie intake.

Don't take my word for it, though. Just check out *any* diet's proposed plan or sample menu and see for yourself. Here are some common ways in which you'll find diets limiting your calories, whether you realize it or not:

◆ "A portion is an amount the size of your fist."

- ◆ "Lower your carbohydrate consumption to 25 grams a day."

- ◆ "You are allowed a daily points range depending on how much you weigh."

- ◆ "Meals should be of normal size and no more."

- ◆ "Limit sweets to 80 calories a day."

- ◆ Sample menu suggestions, such as "bacon, 2 slices" or "tomato juice, 6 ounces." If calories truly weren't an issue and just the *type* of food mattered, why not write "bacon" or "tomato juice" without a specified amount?

Be very aware that cutting back on calories is *the real reason* why any diet succeeds in getting a person to lose weight; the rest is just a lot of hype and gimmicks.

WHAT MOST PEOPLE *DON'T* KNOW ABOUT CALORIES

Since limiting calories is crucial to every successful diet plan, we need to know exactly what these little guys really are. For those of you who think you already know, try my little quiz. True or false—a Whopper with cheese contains about 860 calories?

If you said true, guess what? You're wrong! A Whopper with cheese really has 860,000 calories in it. Puzzled? I'll explain in a minute, but right now, let's try another question. True or false—a Whopper with cheese contains about 860 kilocalories?

If you said *true*, pass go and collect two hundred dollars! While this all might seem a bit confusing, just think of calories as nothing more than *food energy*. Since we need a way to measure this food energy, science has chosen the *kilocalorie* (kcal). Going strictly by the book, one kilocalorie is equal to 1,000 calories. For the more curious and scientific readers who are wondering exactly how much energy a kilocalorie is, it's the amount of heat needed to raise the temperature of one kilogram of water by one degree Celsius.

Now you know why one Whopper with cheese *really* contains 860,000 calories, or 860 kilocalories. While I've chosen to use the word *calorie* throughout this book because most everybody uses it this way as convenient shorthand for *kilocalorie*, know that the proper term is really *kilocalorie*.

WHY SOME THINGS YOU EAT HAVE CALORIES AND OTHERS DON'T

We've established that calories are merely a way to measure the energy from the foods we eat. What's interesting, though, is that not everything you put down the ol' hatch gets used up as energy by your body. In fact, there are actually only *four substances* known to man that can provide the human body with calories. They are:

- ◆ carbohydrates, which have 4 calories per gram

- ◆ fats, which have 9 calories per gram

- ◆ protein, which has 4 calories per gram

- ◆ alcohol, which has 7 calories per gram

Yep, that's it. It makes no difference if you are eating Chinese, Italian, Mexican, or tree bark, for that matter.

Your body will *only* accept these four substances as energy sources and nothing else. While all of them clearly provide your body with calories, you will notice that some of them give you more calories than others. This is why eating foods with a lot of fat in them, such as potato chips, can fatten you up a lot quicker than an apple, which contains mostly carbohydrates. Every gram of *fat* in a food will load you up with 9 calories, while a gram of *carbohydrate* can only give you 4 calories.

Of course, your body also extracts many other things from your food, such as vitamins and minerals, but they *cannot* be used as energy. This is one reason why everybody is always referring to foods as being either a carbohydrate, protein, or fat, or some combination thereof.

IN FIVE MINUTES YOU'RE GOING TO KNOW HOW MANY CALORIES YOU *REALLY* NEED EACH DAY

As you learned from the first chapter, any extra food you eat that your body doesn't use right away gets stored in fat cells called *adipocytes*. Therefore, in order to avoid eating extra calories and having them end up being stored as fat in places where you'd rather not have them, you must know the number of calories your body needs each day. *It is only then that you will know how many calories cause you to gain weight, lose weight, or maintain weight.*

There are two major things a human body "needs" calories for:

◆ *To carry out its vital functions.* This is the number of calories your body uses to sustain life while you're *resting.* For example, even as you lie around, energy is needed to breathe and to keep your heart pumping.

◆ *To fuel its activities.* This is the number of calories your body uses for thinking, for moving around during the day, and for exercising.

Finding out how many calories your body needs to carry out its vital functions and to fuel its activities may sound difficult, but trust me, it's not. All you need is a plain old calculator, a pencil, and a piece of paper, and as long as you're able to push a button, you'll do fine.

Basal Energy Expenditure

Let's start with figuring how many calories you need just to carry out your vital functions. Practically speaking, you could call this the amount of energy you'd burn just lying on the couch all day. A scientist, on the other hand, would call it your *basal energy expenditure* or *BEE.*

Now there are a good number of ways to determine your BEE, but if you walk into any hospital and ask the dietitians which one they most frequently use, the chances are good that most will say the *Harris-Benedict equation.*

The Harris-Benedict equation was derived from rigorous scientific studies done in the early 1900s and has truly stood the test of time. To this day, it remains the most commonly used method for calculating basal energy expenditure for clinical and research purposes. If that makes it sound like a winner, it is. Because it is so popular, some readers may have already heard of it or even used it before—but a word of warning. A 1992 study published in the

Journal of Parenteral and Enteral Nutrition looked at twenty-four published versions of this equation from medical textbooks and compared them to the original one. Many variations were found and, in fact, only *three* references actually cited the equation as it was originally written. Apparently many people have had a lot of trouble copying it correctly.

Whatever the case may be, I have taken much time and care to dig up the *correct* original Harris-Benedict equations (one for men and the other for women). Delivered to you straight from the depths of the medical library's rare-book collection, they are as follows:

Women

EE = 655.0955 + 9.5634*W + 1.8496*H – 4.6756*A

Men

EE = 66.4730 + 13.7516*W + 5.0033*H – 6.7550*A

As you can see, these equations, taken directly from the original study, look kind of, well, *weird*. I'm going to show you step-by-step how to use them correctly.

First you will need to find out your weight *in kilograms:*

weight in kilograms =weight in pounds ÷ 2.2

write down that number _____ = W

Next you will need to find your height *in centimeters:*

height in centimeters = height in inches x 2.54

write down that number _____ = H

Now choose the appropriate section, for women or men, and do the calculations:

For women

1. Begin with 655.0955.

2. Multiply your weight in kilograms, W, by 9.5634.
   Write down that number _____.

3. Multiply your height in centimeters, H, by 1.8496.
   Write down that number _____.

4. Add together the results of steps 1, 2, and 3.
   Write down that number _____.

5. Multiply your age in years, A, by 4.6756.
   Write down that number _____.

6. Subtract the total of step 5 from the total of step 4 to get your BEE (your calorie needs while you're just resting). **Write down that number _____.**

For men

1. Begin with 66.4730.

2. Multiply your weight in kilograms, W, by 13.7516.
   Write down that number _____.

3. Multiply your height in centimeters, H, by 5.0033.
   Write down that number _____.

4. Add together the results from steps 1, 2, and 3.
   Write down that number _____.

5. Multiply your age in years, A, by 6.7550.
   Write down that number _____.

6. Subtract the total of step 5 from the total of step 4 to get your BEE (your calorie needs while you're just resting). **Write down that number _____.**

Typical day-to-day activity level	Activity factor
you are chair-bound or bed-bound	multiply your BEE by 1.2
you do seated work with no option of moving around *and little or no strenuous leisure activity*	multiply your BEE by 1.45
you do seated work with no option of moving around *and significant amounts of sport or strenuous leisure activity for 30–60 minutes, 4–5 times a week*	multiply your BEE by 1.75
you do seated work with discretion and requirement to move around *but little or no strenuous leisure activity*	multiply your BEE by 1.65
you do seated work with discretion and requirement to move around *but significant amounts of sport or strenuous leisure activity for 30–60 minutes, 4–5 times a week*	multiply your BEE by 1.95
you do a lot of standing work, such as a housewife or shop assistant, *and little or no strenuous leisure activity*	multiply your BEE by 1.85
you do a lot of standing work, such as housewife or shop assistant, *and significant amounts of sport or strenuous leisure activity for 30–60 minutes, 4–5 times a week*	multiply your BEE by 2.15
you do strenuous work or have highly active leisure activities	multiply your BEE by 2.2

Adapted from Black A. E., W. A. Coward, T. J. Cole, and A. M. Prentice. 1996. Human energy expenditure in affluent societies: An analysis of 574 doubly-labelled water measurements. *European Journal of Clinical Nutrition* 50, 72–92.

Applying Activity Factors

Now you know how many calories you need just to keep your body alive while you're resting. However, since we do move around and don't just lie still in one place all day long, we must take this into account when figuring out how many total calories we need in a day. This is done quite easily by taking your BEE (the number you got for step 6) and multiplying it by one of the activity factors described in the table on page 58. Review the table and choose the category that best describes your your typical day-to-day activity level.

BEE x activity factor = the number of calories you need each day, or your baseline calorie needs.

Write down that number _____.

Here is a real life example of how calculating the equation should look, using myself as the guinea pig:

Jim is thirty-eight years old, 6' 1", and weights 175 pounds. He is a physical therapist working at a large teaching hospital, where he treats outpatients with various body aches and pains. He also spends time each day on the floors helping people to stand and walk again. Leisure activities and exercise include walking for thirty minutes four to five times a week, plus lifting weights for forty-five minutes twice a week.

First I'll need to convert my height to centimeters and my weight to kilograms:

Weight: 175 pounds ÷ 2.2 = 80 kilograms
Height: 6' 1" = 73 inches; 73 x 2.54 = 185 centimeters

Next, I use the equation for men:

1. Begin with 66.4730	66.4730
2. Multiply your weight in kilograms (as you already figured out above) by 13.7516.	80 x 13.7516 = 1,100
3. Multiply your height in centimeters (as you already figured out above) by 5.0033.	185 x 5.0033 = 926
4. Add together the results from steps 1, 2, and 3.	66.4730 + 1,100 + 926 = 2,092
5. Multiply your age by 6.7550.	38 x 6.7550 = 257
6. Subtract the total of step 5 from the total of step 4 to get your BEE (your calorie needs while resting).	2,092 – 257 = 1,835 **Jim's BEE is 1,835 calories.**

As you can see, I need 1,835 calories just to keep my body running. Now we add in the calories I'll need for moving around and exercising by multiplying the BEE by the activity factor that best fits my lifestyle:

BEE x Activity Factor = how many *total* calories Jim needs in a day (his baseline calorie needs).

1,835 x 1.95 = 3,578. Jim needs 3,578 calories a day.

Congratulations! By using some of the most well-researched equations known to man, you have just figured out your baseline calories needs, which is how many calories you *really* need in one day. While it is only an *estimate*, keep in mind that probably the only way to get more accurate than this would be for you to go through formal testing using fancy equipment. However, since the vast majority of doctors and nutritionists figure out energy requirements using the Harris-Benedict equation, it will suit our needs as well.

HOW TO TAKE THE GUESSWORK OUT OF LOSING WEIGHT

Now that you know your baseline calorie needs, you're in the driver's seat. Why? Because if you know that you've eaten *more* calories than you need in a day, you can expect to gain weight—and that means it's time to make adjustments and get back on track. On the other hand, if you know you've eaten *fewer* calories than you need in a day, then you can look forward to losing weight—and you're another day closer to reaching your goal. But how will you know if you've eaten too much or too little over a day's time?

Simple. By keeping track of how many calories you've eaten during the day. Yes, this does mean you will have to use a little elbow grease in the beginning. But let me tell you that keeping track of your calories only gets easier and easier with time. In fact, in just a matter of weeks you will more than likely develop what I call "calorie sense" and be able to just glance at the foods you regularly eat and know

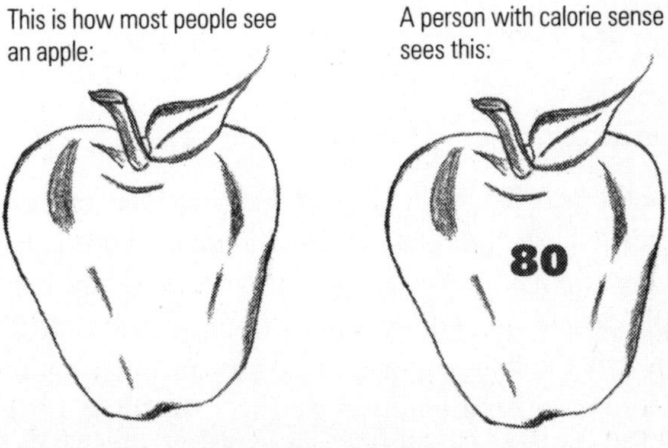

This is how most people see an apple:

A person with calorie sense sees this:

80

Figure 4.1. Calorie sense.

about how many calories they contain. Figure 4.1 is an example of how someone with calorie sense sees things.

Developing your calorie sense is bound to happen, because once you've looked up the calories for a particular food a time or two or know how many calories are in an entrée at your favorite restaurant, the hard work is over. From that point on, you'll *always* know how many calories are in the foods you regularly eat. This does *not* mean that all the fun is going to be taken out of eating. Instead, think of it as gaining an awareness of how much energy is in the foods you eat *and* finding a balance at mealtime. Know, too, that with this kind of awareness also comes a sense of freedom. Why? Because knowing how many calories you've eaten in a day will let you know right then and there whether you can expect to gain, maintain, or lose weight. No more *wondering* if your diet plan will really work or not. Practically speaking, you're taking the guesswork out of everything.

Now, before you slam this book shut thinking you've already heard all about calorie counting, just remember what you read at the beginning of the chapter:

> The unavoidable truth is that *all* successful weight-loss diets work for the exact same reason: They give your body a smaller supply of calories (energy) to run on, which forces you to use up your fat stores.

In the last chapter, I cited no fewer than three scientific studies published in peer-reviewed journals showing that diet *makeup* has absolutely nothing to do with how much weight people lose. For example, as long as everybody in a study eats the same number of calories a day, *all* subjects will lose a similar amount of weight, even though some subjects may eat a high-*carbohydrate* diet, and others a high-*fat* diet. And in the beginning of this chapter, you saw many examples of how weight-loss diets all have one thing in common—they limit calories.

I say it's time to end any confusion or misconceptions here and now. When the smoke clears and the dust settles, *limiting the total number of calories you eat in a day is what makes any weight-loss diet work*. Therefore, if you're gonna lose weight by dieting, it's best to keep track of your calories one way or another!

Sure, you could just start eating a little less food each day without knowing how many calories you've eaten, hoping that you will lose some weight. But that's exactly what you'd be doing—*hoping*. Talk about playing a game of roulette. Maybe you've cut your calories enough to get below your daily calorie needs, maybe you haven't. If you do happen to cut your calories low enough to lose weight, will you really have any idea how much you can expect to lose? Probably not. And how long will you keep losing weight? You won't have a clue. On the other hand, the person who *does* assess her or his daily calorie intake knows the answers to *all* of these questions.

Know, too, that people often make keeping track of calories a much bigger deal than it really is. In reality, it takes *mere minutes* a day, requires no fancy equipment, and is no harder than adding or pushing buttons on a calculator—skills everyone learned in grade school. And these days, *counting calories is easier than ever*. Why? Because the United States government has made it easy for you. Does Figure 4.2 on the next page look familiar?

Of course it does! That's because since 1994, food manufacturers have been required *by law* to put nutrition labels like the one above on practically everything you can buy in the grocery store. This is very good news because it means that most of the foods you buy and eat *must* have the number of calories they contain printed right on the label. And how handy is that?

For the few foods that are not required by law to carry a nutrition label (alcohol and most raw foods, i.e., fresh fruits, fresh vegetables, fresh fish, fresh meats), just buy a calorie counter. They are under ten dollars, and I know of some that even include listings for the foods from over one hundred fast-food chains and restaurants! So, you can see that finding the number of calories in foods these days is far from rocket science.

To further help you keep track of calories, I've

Nutrition Facts

Serving Size About 5 biscuits (51g/1.8 oz.)
Servings per Container   About 11

Amount Per Serving	Cereal	Cereal with ½ Cup Vitamins A & D Skim Milk
Calories	180	220
Calories from Fat	10	10

	% Daily Value **	
Total Fat 1.0g*	**2 %**	**2 %**
Saturated Fat 0g	**0 %**	**0 %**
Monounsaturated 0g		
Polyunsaturated 0.5g		
Cholesterol 0mg	**0 %**	**0 %**
Sodium 0mg	**0 %**	**3 %**
Potassium 170mg	**5 %**	**11 %**
Total Carbohydrate 41g	**14 %**	**16 %**
Dietary Fiber 5g	**20 %**	**20 %**
Sugars 10g		
Other Carbohydrate 26g		
Protein 5g		

Vitamin A	0 %	4 %
Vitamin C	0 %	2 %
Calcium	0 %	15 %
Iron	80 %	80 %

*Amount in cereal. One half cup skim milk contributes an additional 40 calories, 65mg sodium, 6g total carbohydrate (6g sugars), and 4g protein.
** Percent Daily Values are based on a 2,000 calorie diet. Your daily values may be higher or lower depending on your calorie needs:

	Calories	2,000	2,500
Total Fat	Less than	65g	80g
Sat. Fat	Less than	20g	25g
Cholesterol	Less than	300mg	300mg
Sodium	Less than	2,400mg	2,400mg
Potassium		3,500mg	3,500mg
Total Carbohydrate		300g	375g
Dietary Fiber		25g	30g

Figure 4.2. A nutrition label.

provided you with a handy calorie-intake card that you can use each day. It looks like this (see page 65):

Su M T W T F Sa (circle one)   Calories per food item

Breakfast _____   _____

_____   _____

_____   _____

_____   _____

_____   _____

Total for breakfast   _____

Lunch _____   _____

_____   _____

_____   _____

_____   _____

Total for lunch   _____

Dinner _____   _____

_____   _____

_____   _____

_____   _____

_____   _____

_____   _____

_____   _____

Total for dinner   _____

Snacks _____   _____

_____   _____

_____   _____

_____   _____

Total for snacks   _____

Baseline calorie needs _____ Today's calorie intake   _____

Calorie-Intake Card

You will find more blank calorie-intake cards in the Appendix at the end of the book, so you can make copies to use each day. All you have to do is take a minute or two after each meal to jot down the foods you have just eaten as well as the calorie content from any nutrition labels. If you don't have the number of calories right in front of you, that's fine; it only means you'll have to take a few minutes later on to look them up and write them in. At the end of the day, finish by totaling the calories for each individual meal (i.e., breakfast, lunch, etc.), and then, going down the right-hand column, add up the totals from all your meals and snacks to get your total calorie intake for the day.

The number you got from doing the calculations in the preceding section (Harris-Benedict equation times appropriate activity factor) goes on the line labeled "Baseline calorie needs." When all is said and done, if you find that the number you write on the line labeled "Today's calorie intake" is *more* than your "Baseline calorie needs," that means your body will store the extra calories and you'll be gaining weight. On the other hand, if "Today's calorie intake" is *less* than your "Baseline calorie needs," that means you have successfully created a calorie deficit and have forced your body to use up some of its stored fat—so look forward to losing some weight!

All of this—writing down the foods you have eaten and adding up the calories—should take you no more than minutes a day. Just make the time to fill out the card and move on; the rewards are waiting for you.

Don't be surprised if after a week or two of doing this you find yourself looking at fewer and fewer nutrition labels. Because we have a tendency to eat many of the same foods over and over, you will soon start to become quite familiar with how many calories exist in the foods you regularly eat. Only occasionally will you have to look up a food item you haven't eaten before or haven't eaten recently.

I've said from the start that this book is every bit as *practical* as it is evidence based, so let's look at an example of how easy and efficient it is to actually use the calorie-intake card while going about a typical day. Once again, I'll be the guinea pig.

I stumble down the stairs about 6:30 A.M.—I'm definitely *not* a morning person. My wife, a cardiac rehab nurse, is long gone by that time, having to get up at 4:30 to be at work by 6:00. As I head to the kitchen, my son is also up, ready to catch the bus to high school. I have a quick bowl of cereal with him, and then it's time to get my eleven-year-old daughter up and off to school.

After fighting traffic for forty-five minutes, I arrive at work about 8:00. I usually see outpatients all morning—many times a new patient every thirty minutes. Being this busy, I don't usually have time to stop and think about being hungry, but if I do, I eat a granola bar that I keep in my desk.

Finally it's lunchtime. By now, I'm good and ready to sit down, having been on my feet all morning long. I usually run down to the cafeteria to get a diet soda and then sit at my desk to eat. Today I have a peanut butter and jelly sandwich, an easy-open can of pineapple, and a prepackaged container of flavored applesauce.

It's about 1:00 in the afternoon now, which is when I start wandering the floors of the hospital to treat my inpatients. This can be quite challenging, as most of my patients, carrying a wide variety of diagnoses from hip replacements to liver transplants, have been *very* sick and in bed for literally weeks. My job is to get them up and moving again. During this time, I can take breaks in between patients if I feel the need to, and I often get in a quick snack—usually consisting of a cup of hot chocolate and a small package of graham crackers—by raiding one of the hospital floor's kitchens.

My workday ends at around 4:30, which means I get home (provided there are no traffic accidents) at 5:30. My wife usually beats me home, and tonight she has decided to barbecue chicken out on the grill. In addition, I have a baked potato with no-calorie spray butter, corn on the cob with no-calorie spray butter, and a salad. I wash it all down with several glasses of calorie-free lemonade.

After finishing dinner, cleaning up, and helping the kids with homework, my wife and I go for a twenty-five-minute walk around the neighborhood. Tonight I felt like I needed a snack after the walk and gulped down a glass of milk mixed with Ovaltine. After writing for about an hour and a half or so, it's off to bed.

When all was said and done, at the end of the day my filled-in calorie-intake card looked like the one on page 69. Look like a lot of work? Not really. Most of the work had already been done for me, thanks to the nutrition labels. Here's how I did it, *in minutes:*

I folded my calorie card in half and stuck it into my pocket before leaving for work. Every time I finished eating something, I jotted it down. Because of nutrition labels, I was able to quickly figure out *on the spot* how many calories there were in most of the foods I ate and decided to note this in parentheses. For instance, you'll see the first thing I

Su M T W T F Sa (circle one)   Calories per food item

		Calories per food item
Breakfast	bowl of cereal w/milk	340
	Total for breakfast	340
Lunch	peanut butter/jelly sandwich	410
	applesauce	90
	pineapple	50
	Total for lunch	550
Dinner	3 drumsticks	288
	salad (w/ 2 T. dressing)	85
	2 ears of corn	160
	baked potato	156
	Total for dinner	689
Snacks	granola bar	180
	hot chocolate	100
	graham crackers	60
	Ovaltine	180
	Total for snacks	520

Baseline calorie needs __3,578__ Today's calorie intake __2,099__

Calorie-Intake Card

ate was a bowl of cereal. To figure out how many calories I got from eating just this bowl of cereal, I quickly scanned the nutrition label on the side of the cereal box and looked for the number of calories. The label said "120." Okay, that's nice, but *how much cereal* is equal to 120 calories?

No problem, just look at the *serving size*—it's also on the nutrition label and tells you exactly how much cereal is equal to 120 calories. In this case, the nutrition label on my box of cereal said that one cup of cereal is equal to 120 calories (you'll soon be noticing that every serving size on a nutrition label is in commonly used measurements such as tablespoons or cups to make it easy on you).

See what I mean? Just by scanning the nutrition label for a few seconds, I was able to tell that one cup of cereal is equal to 120 calories. The only thing left now is figuring out how much cereal I actually poured in my bowl and ate. Since I normally just fill 'er up and eat without first measuring the cereal, I really have no idea how many cups there are in a bowl. So I grab a measuring cup and pour two cups of cereal into my bowl—that seems about right. From now on, *I'll always know* that I eat about two cups of cereal in the morning, which is equal to 240 calories (one cup equals 120 calories, so two cups equals 240). But don't forget about the milk.

I have to do the same thing with the milk that I did with the cereal. Looking on the side of the milk jug at the nutrition label, I saw 100 calories. But 100 calories is how much milk? A quick scan for the serving size shows one cup. This means one cup of milk equals 100 calories. Once again, I'm not quite sure how much milk I normally use, so I have to do my little test (for the first and last time unless I just forget). I poured one measuring cup of milk in my cereal, and it looked like the usual amount. Once again, I now know I eat about one cup of milk every day with my cereal, which is 100 calories.

And for the grand calorie total for a bowl of cereal, I simply add the 240 cereal calories to the 100 milk calories in my head and I've got…Jim's 340-calorie breakfast!

While this all reads rather slow, in reality it took me only *seconds* to scan the nutrition labels and no more than a minute to measure out the servings with a measuring cup. After that, I just wrote down the food item on my calorie card, added up the numbers in my head, and jotted them down on the calorie card. Done.

Throughout the day, I continued to write down all of the foods I ate. On this particular day, I was able to get the number of calories of every food item I ate from the nutrition labels except for *three* (which I looked up later that evening in my calorie counter).

For readers who are more visually oriented, there's the breakdown in table form on page 72 of how I got the numbers you see on my calorie-intake card. Please note that you *do not* have to write everything out as I have. This table is included *only* to serve as an example of how to take the information from the nutrition label and figure out how many calories you have eaten.

As mentioned earlier, keeping track of your daily calorie intake is something that only gets easier. It starts out with writing things down on the calorie card and doing a few measurements now and then with common household items such as cups and tablespoons. In time, and through repetition, you will find yourself measuring and calculating less and less because you will come to know how many calories are in a glass of milk or a ham sandwich by merely

Food item I wrote down	Serving size listed on the nutrition label or calorie counter	# of calories per serving, as listed on the food label	How much food I ate	# of calories I ate
bowl of cereal	1 cup	120 calories/cup	2 cups	240 calories
	1 cup of milk	100 calories/cup	1 cup	100 calories
granola bar	2 bars per package	180 calories/2 bars	2 bars	180 calories
peanut butter/jelly sandwich	2 tablespoons peanut butter	190 calories/2 tablespoons	2 tablespoons	190 calories
	1 tablespoon grape jelly	50 calories/tablespoon	2 tablespoons	100 calories
	1 slice of bread	60 calories/slice	2 slices	120 calories
pineapple	1 can	50 calories/can	1 can	50 calories
applesauce	1 container	90 calories/container	1 container	90 calories
hot chocolate	1 packet	100 calories/packet	1 packet	100 calories
graham crackers	1 packet	60 calories/packet	1 packet	60 calories
3 chicken drumsticks	1 drumstick	76 calories/drumstick	3 drumsticks	228 calories
	2 tablespoons barbecue sauce	60 calories/2 tablespoons	2 tablespoons	60 calories
baked potato	1 potato	156 calories/potato	1 potato	156 calories
2 ears of corn	1 corn on the cob	80 calories/cob	2 cobs	160 calories
salad	2 cups	15 calories/2 cups	2 cups	15 calories
	2 tablespoons salad dressing	70 calories/2 tablespoons	2 tablespoons	70 calories
glass of Ovaltine	1 cup milk	100 calories/cup	1 cup	100 calories
	4 tablespoons Ovaltine	80 calories/4 tablespoons	4 tablespoons	80 calories

"eyeballing" them—something I refer to as "calorie sense." Ultimately, when you have reached your ideal body weight and no longer have to adjust your daily calorie intake, your calorie sense will more than likely give you an idea of just how much food you can eat each day to maintain your weight *without* having to write things down. At that point, you will have made a lifestyle change that's good *for the rest of your life*.

DON'T CUT CALORIES UNTIL YOU'VE READ THIS FIRST

Now that you know how many calories you need in a day and you have a handy way of keeping track of them, the last issue to consider is what combination of fats, carbohydrates, and proteins should make up those calories?

Where do you suppose I could get the answer to such a question? Does it come from the results of one or two scientific studies? Nope. Relying on just one or two studies to get your nutritional information is actually a terrible mistake. It's what the *majority* of studies say that's really important. In other words, we want to look at trends in the literature, not just the results of an isolated study or two.

Yes, I admit it's hard to know who to believe at times without having a degree in research. I remember one time reading the diet chapter of a best-selling fitness book that almost seemed to warn its readers about "experts." In fact, the book even pointed out that a lot of "experts" are actually more confused than the people they are trying to help!

Well, I have a news flash. The experts are *not* confused, although they do make good targets for people who are trying to sell you something.

The truth is that while differences of opinion *do* exist among experts in the field of nutrition (as in any field), the majority of experts can still all sit down together and agree on a standard for people's energy and nutrient intakes. I can prove it because such events have been going on for quite some time now. In the United States, the results of such gatherings are known as the *recommended dietary allowances*, or RDA. Here are some facts about the RDA that I'm betting a lot of people aren't even aware of:

- ◆ The RDA are intended for *healthy* people.

- ◆ The RDA are based on the available scientific research.

- ◆ The RDA have been around for over sixty years and continue to be revised periodically in order to keep them up-to-date.

- ◆ Although this work is funded by the government, the committee that sets the RDA is made up of scientists from different specialties.

- ◆ The RDA are *recommended* dietary allowances, not *required* dietary allowances. In other words, they are suggested average daily nutrient intake levels sufficient to meet the nutrient requirements of nearly all healthy people.

Although the RDA may lack the charisma and charm of fad diets, nothing can take away the fact that they are one of the most updated, well-researched, and evidence-backed set of nutritional recommendations on the face of the planet. And that's *exactly* what we want when it comes to our health!

Now let's have a look at some of the current recommended dietary allowances for fats, carbohydrates, and proteins. The majority of the following information has been adapted from *Report Brief: Dietary Reference Intakes for Energy, Carbohydrate, Fiber, Fat, Fatty Acids, Cholesterol, Protein, and Amino Acids* (National Academy of Sciences, 2002). I suggest comparing these recommendations to your own diet to see how adequate it is.

Fats

About 20–35 percent of your diet should be made up of fats. Be aware, however, that not all fats are created equal. There are, in fact, four major kinds of fats in the foods you eat, two being the "good" kind, and two being the "bad" kind:

◆ Monounsaturated fats are "good" fats because they can lower your cholesterol levels, which reduces your risk of heart disease. Some sources include olive oil, canola oil, peanut oil, and avocados.

◆ Polyunsaturated fats are also "good" fats because they, too, can lower your cholesterol levels, which reduces your risk of heart disease. You need two types: alpha-linolenic acid and linoleic acid. Some sources of alpha-linolenic acid include soybean oil, canola oil, flaxseed oil, and fish oils. Some sources of linoleic acid include nuts, seeds, soybean oil, safflower oil, and corn oil.

◆ Saturated fats are "bad" fats because they can raise your cholesterol levels, which increases your risk of heart disease. Some foods that contain saturated fats include meats, bakery items, and full-fat dairy products.

◆ Trans fatty acids are "bad" fats, as they too can raise your cholesterol levels, which increases your risk of heart disease. Some foods that contain trans fatty acids include many cookies, crackers, cakes, French fries, fried onion rings, and donuts.

There are no recommended dietary allowances set for saturated fats and trans fatty acids because they have no known beneficial role in preventing chronic diseases and are therefore not needed at any level in your diet. Practically speaking, this means eat as little of them as possible. Nutrition labels can help you out with this, as the amount of saturated fat in a food (listed in grams) is required to be listed.

On the other hand, people *must* get two kinds of polyunsaturated fatty acids, alpha-linolenic acid (an omega-3 fatty acid) and linoleic acid (an omega-6 fatty acid), from the foods they eat, because the human body cannot make them. (For that reason, they're called *essential fatty acids.*) The chances of your having a deficiency of one of these if you live in the United States is extremely rare. But just so you have all the facts, the tables below list the adequate intakes for these essential fatty acids:

Linoleic acid

Males		Females	
Age	Grams/day	Age	Grams/day
19–30	17	19–30	12
31–50	17	31–50	12
50–70	14	50–70	11

Alpha-linolenic acid

Males		**Females**	
Age	Grams/day	Age	Grams/day
19–30	1.6	19–30	1.1
31–50	1.6	31–50	1.1
50–70	1.6	50–70	1.1

Carbohydrates

Forty-five to 65 percent of your diet should be made up of carbohydrates. The major types are sugars and starches. Here is a list to give you an idea of which is which:

Sources of starches	**Sources of sugars**
grains	fruits
pasta	juices
rice	soft drinks
potatoes	candy
breads	desserts
corn	fruit drinks

To stay healthy, the RDA say that each day adults need to eat *at least* 130 grams of digestible carbohydrates (as opposed to fiber, which is also a carbohydrate but which passes through the digestive tract undigested). Most people, however, usually exceed this amount. Once again, use the nutrition label to easily find out how many grams you're eating in a day.

Protein

As you read in Chapter 3, people have been recorded as dying when they have cut their calories and failed to get the proper protein requirements (recall the very low calorie diets of the 1970s and 80s). Proteins repair or replace worn-out tissues and are the major structural components of every cell in your body. As you have probably guessed by now, protein is one nutrient not to be neglected while dieting!

Ten to 35 percent of your diet should be made up of protein. The RDA for men and women is listed as 0.8 grams of protein for every kilogram of body weight. Here's how you can quite easily figure out how much protein you need every day:

First you will need to find how much you weigh in kilograms:

weight in kilograms = weight in pounds ÷ 2.2

Write down that number _____.

Next, simply multiply your weight in kilograms by 0.8:

your weight in kilograms x 0.8 = how many grams of protein you need each day

And here's a real-life example, using yours truly once again:

175 pounds ÷ 2.2 = 80 kilograms

80 kilograms x 0.8 = 64

It is recommended that Jim get 64 grams of protein a day.

What could be easier? And at risk of sounding like a broken record, just add up the grams of protein on the nutrition labels or from your calorie counter for a given day to see how close you're coming to meeting these levels.

HOW TO CALCULATE THE PERCENTAGES OF FATS, CARBOHYDRATES, AND PROTEINS IN YOUR DIET

As you have noticed, for each of the individual nutrients we've discussed so far—fats, carbohydrates, and proteins— I have told you the recommended percentages of each that should make up your diet. For instance, it is recommended that protein should make up around 10 to 35 percent of your diet. That's good and fine, but how does one know if 10 to 35 percent of their diet is really made up of protein?

By running a few totals and doing two simple math equations. But hold on, this is not something you have to do every day. It is another tool I'm going to let you know about so every now and then you can spot-check your own diet and see how it stacks up against the recommendations. Here's what you do:

First you have to know how many grams of each nutrient you have eaten in a day. Do this by simply reading the nutrition labels or the listings in your calorie counter and then adding up the totals for the day of that particular nutrient. For example, I looked at the nutrition labels and found that I ate a total of 70 grams of protein on Monday.

Now that I know how many grams of protein I have eaten, I need to know how many calories this is equal to. Since there are 4 calories in every gram of protein, I just multiply the 70 grams by 4:

70 grams of protein x 4 calories per gram of protein = 280 calories

Jim got 280 calories from protein on Monday.

All that's left to do now is to divide the number of protein calories (280) by the total number of calories I ate on Monday (2,099). I got this number from my calorie card. The last step looks like this:

280 protein calories ÷ 2,099 total daily calories = 0.13, or 13 percent

Thirteen percent of Jim's diet that day was made up of protein.

Looks like I did well as far as protein is concerned. I am aiming for the recommended 10 to 35 percent and ended up with 13 percent that day. Not bad—I'll try to spot-check it again every so often to see how I'm doing.

The same calculation can be used to find out your carbohydrate percentage, because carbs and protein both contain 4 calories per gram. Simply add up the number of grams of carbohydrates you ate in a day (325 in my example), and multiply that number by four. Then take the result and divide it by your total daily calories to get the percentage of calories from carbohydrates you ate that day. For instance:

325 grams of carbohydrates x 4 calories per gram of carbohydrate = 1,300 calories

1,300 carb calories ÷ 2,099 total daily calories = 0.62, or 62 percent

Sixty-two percent of Jim's diet that day was made up of carbohydrates.

For fats, it's just a hair different because fats have 9 calories per gram instead of the 4 calories per gram that proteins and carbohydrates have. Therefore, simply add up the number of grams of fat you ate in a day (59 in my example), and multiply that number by nine. Then take the result and divide it by your daily total calories in order to get the percentage of calories from fat you ate that day. It will go like this:

> 59 grams of fat x 9 calories per gram of fat = 531 calories

> 531 fat calories ÷ 2,099 total daily calories = 0.25, or 25 percent

> Twenty-five percent of Jim's diet that day was made up of fats.

As I said earlier, this is *not* something you have to do every day or even every week. And it certainly isn't something you must do in order to lose weight. It's merely a good tool to pull out once in awhile to make sure you're eating a nutritionally balanced diet.

A COMMON MISTAKE PEOPLE MAKE WHILE DIETING

Now you know how to figure out how many calories you need to start losing weight. You also know that roughly 45–65 percent of those calories should come from carbohydrates, 20–35 percent from fats, and 10–35 percent from protein. So you're good to go, right?

Well, you *could* run into a problem if I left it at that. While you certainly would lose weight if you followed only this advice, you might also be eating *very unhealthily*. Let me illustrate:

Jim figured out he needs 3,578 calories a day.

It is recommended that 45–65 percent of those calories should come from carbohydrates.

Therefore, about 1,610–2,326 of the 3,578 calories should come from carbohydrates.

Taking all this advice to heart, Jim decides to eat 2,300 calories worth of Twizzlers (a carbohydrate) one day, stays well within his carbohydrate calorie limit, and successfully loses weight.

The problem? Sure, Jim *is* losing weight. But he's also losing a lot more than that—things such as vitamins, minerals, and fiber, nutrients that his body needs *every day* to function properly and stay healthy!

While this book has pointed out the fact that the only substances that contain calories are fats, carbohydrates, protein, and alcohol, does that mean nutrients like vitamins, minerals, and fiber don't matter, since they contain *no* calories? Of course not. They may not enter into the weight-loss equation at all, but we all know how important they are to our health.

So just how *do* you make sure to get plenty of these important nutrients? Simple. Since different foods contain different nutrients, and no one food can give you all the nutrients you need, *choose from a wide variety of foods.* Remember the five basic food groups?

- The bread, cereal, rice, and pasta group

- The fruit group

- The vegetable group

- ◆ The meat, poultry, fish, dry beans, eggs, and nuts group

- ◆ The milk, yogurt, and cheese group

Certainly in the above example Jim would have been much better off nutritionally if he had chosen to eat 2,300 calories worth of fruits, vegetables, and pasta *instead of* 2,300 calories worth of Twizzlers in order to get his recommended amount of carbohydrates.

The bottom line? Make sure it's the *calories* you're cutting from your diet, not the nutrition. Eating a wide variety of foods is an important part of getting all the nutrients your body needs.

HOW TO GET STARTED... TODAY!

Okay. By this point you've probably got monounsaturated fats and gram-counting coming out of your ears! It's true we've covered a lot of stuff in this chapter, but now I'm going to show you how to pull it all together with the least amount of effort and put the diet strategy into action.

First, start by finding out how many calories you need each day by using the Harris-Benedict equation and the appropriate activity factor. Write this number in the line labeled "Baseline calorie needs" on your calorie card.

Next, use the calorie card to keep track of how many calories you eat each day, using food nutrition labels and a calorie counter as needed. Add up the total number of calories at the end of each day, and write the number in the line labeled "Today's calorie intake" on your calorie card.

Now it's time to start getting rid of that body fat. To lose weight with a diet strategy, you must create a calorie shortage by eating *fewer* calories than your body needs. For instance, if you've calculated that you need 2,000 calories a day by using the Harris-Benedict equation and the appropriate activity factor, and you eat 2,500 calories, you *will not* lose weight; in fact you've gone way over your calorie needs and will actually *gain* weight. On the other hand, if you need 2,000 calories a day and eat 1,500, you will definitely lose weight; your body now has to rely on its fat stores for energy since you were such a cheapskate with the food. In terms of your calorie card, you'll always want "Today's calorie intake" to be *less* than "Baseline calorie needs" in order to lose weight.

Let's move on to predicting how much weight you will lose and how fast you'll lose it. This all depends on how many calories you cut *below* what your body needs each day. It's a fact that you must burn 3,500 calories to lose a pound of body fat, and it's a fact that there are seven days in a week. Therefore, to lose one pound a week, you would need to eat 500 calories *less* each day than your daily calorie needs, since $7 \times 500 = 3,500$. To lose two pounds a week by just dieting, you would need to eat 1,000 calories *less* each day than your daily calorie needs, since $7 \times 1,000 = 7,000$, and since it takes 7,000 calories to burn two pounds of body fat.

Wow! A thousand calories is *a lot* to cut back on each day. For that reason, I don't recommended that you try to lose any more than one to two pounds a week at the most by dieting alone. I *highly* suggest using the diet part of the Dianex Strategy to aim for losing about a half pound to a pound per week and the exercise part of the strategy to lose any additional weight. (After all, this is a diet strategy, not a *famine* strategy!) Losing a half pound in a week means eating 250 calories a day less than your daily baseline calorie needs. Losing a pound in a week means eating 500 calories a day less than your daily baseline calorie needs.

Now don't shoot me, but as your weight goes down, so do your body's calorie needs. Practically speaking, this means that as you weigh less and less, you have to eat less and less because your body needs fewer calories to keep itself running. To keep tabs on this, I suggest refiguring your baseline calorie needs about *once a month* using the Harris-Benedict equation and the appropriate activity factor to see if your baseline calorie needs have in fact changed. If they have, make sure to put your new baseline calorie needs in the appropriate line on your calorie card.

In the not so distant future, when you have reached your ideal body weight, you can easily find out how many calories you need each day to maintain this weight. Simply calculate your baseline calorie needs at that time using the Harris-Benedict equation and appropriate activity factor. If, for example, you find your baseline calorie needs at your ideal body weight to be 2,000 a day, and you eat 2,000 calories a day, you will maintain your current weight. At that point, you can choose to either continue tracking your calories each day with the calorie card or just spot-check them every few days and make adjustments as you need to. In reality, though, I'm betting a lot of readers will probably be so acutely aware of the calorie content of foods by this time that their calorie sense will be able to give them a good idea of just how much food they can eat each day *without* having to write things down. And that's exactly the kind of lifestyle change we're shooting for!

Chapter 4 in a Nutshell

◆ A calorie is just the way we measure food energy.

◆ All weight-loss diets have one thing in common: They limit calories.

◆ All successful weight-loss diets work for the same reason: They limit calories.

◆ Your body can only get calories from carbohydrates, fats, protein, and alcohol.

◆ A good way to estimate how many calories you need in a day (your baseline calorie needs) is to use the Harris-Benedict equation and an appropriate activity factor. Knowing your baseline calorie needs lets you know how many calories will cause you to gain weight, lose weight, or remain the same.

◆ To lose weight, you must eat fewer calories than your baseline calorie needs.

◆ Aim for a one-half to one pound weight loss each week by using the diet part of the Dianex Strategy. This is done by eating 250 to 500 calories a day less than your baseline calorie needs. I don't recommended that you try to lose any more than one to two pounds a week, at the most, by just dieting.

◆ Keeping track of your calories takes all the guesswork out of dieting because it lets you know right away if you're eating the right amount to successfully lose weight. Calorie cards and nutrition labels are an easy and inexpensive way to do this.

◆ Compare your diet to the RDAs' evidence-backed guidelines. Doing so will help ensure that you are eating healthily.

◆ To meet your body's nutritional needs, eat a wide variety of foods from the five basic food groups every day.

5

The Exercise Strategy

If you don't want to be where you've always been,
change what you've always done.

A marathon is a long way to run. In fact, it's exactly 26.2 miles. How much weight do you think you would lose if you could run a marathon, right now?

Well, the exercise-physiology books tell me that finishing a 26.2-mile marathon requires an energy expenditure of about 100 calories a mile. This means if a person did indeed use up 100 calories a mile and ran the full 26.2 miles, they would burn off about 2,620 calories. Now this may not sound too bad, until you realize that this is actually *far less* than the 3,500-calorie deficit you need in order to burn just one pound of body fat!

The point here is not to make a case against exercising, but rather to put things into their proper perspective. It takes a heckuva lot of exercise to lose weight, and if you're a woman, you may not even lose weight at all by exercise only, according to multiple randomized controlled trials.

As the scientific literature also tells us, an exercise strategy is most effective for weight loss when combined with a diet strategy. Keep this in mind the next time you're at the bookstore and see a fitness book that promises a fantastic-looking body with just minutes of exercise in the morning or some special workout technique. In reality, the chances are quite good that any weight-loss results you get would really be due to the fact that the exercise program was combined with a diet plan, *not* the few minutes of exercise or the revolutionary new workout technique. Certainly it's much easier to see things for what they really are when you know what to look for.

Having said that, I figure that by this time *everybody* knows that exercise is good for them, that it can help them lose weight, and the more the better. After spending years teaching therapeutic exercises to patients, I have identified four major obstacles that keep most people from consistently exercising. They are

- ◆ a lack of motivation
- ◆ a lack of time
- ◆ a dislike of exercise
- ◆ no access to exercise equipment

The first, and perhaps most critical, obstacle, motivation, has already been discussed in Chapter 2. Thus, we have three obstacles left to tackle.

While I could just whip out my pom-poms and tell you to get off the couch, find the time to work out, and quit making excuses, the truth is that I honestly feel that these are legitimate barriers that keep many, many people from exercising. Therefore, if I realistically expect to get anybody to consistently exercise over the long run, I darn well better find an exercise strategy that will fit into a busy schedule, will appeal to those who hate exercise, and can be done without equipment. Question is, does one exist?

Well, believe it or not, you're just pages away from learning about one. Not only is there an exercise strategy out there that meets *all* of these requirements, but it has also been proven to be *just as effective* when stacked up against traditional exercises you've probably tried in the past. And, as always, I'll be showing you the randomized controlled trials that back it up, just so you can rest assured that *this* exercise strategy can really get you where you want to be.

GIVE YOUR SNEAKERS AND THE GYM A REST—I'M ONLY GOING TO ASK YOU TO DO ONE THING

Unlike a lot of people who fall asleep at the sight of a research article, I just love digging around in the scientific literature and reading studies. Even after being into research for well over a decade, few things give me greater pleasure than researching a topic and getting to the bottom of things, especially when I know I can bring the information to a lot of people who would otherwise have never known about it.

Some time ago, on one such adventure in the medical library, I stumbled across an article that went totally against the traditional idea of exercise I had been taught in physical-therapy school. Published in a January 1999 issue of *The Journal of the American Medical Association*, the study went like this:

> Forty obese women were randomly assigned to one of two exercise groups (Andersen, 1999). The first exercise group participated in step-aerobics classes,

while the second group was told to increase their levels of moderate-intensity physical activity by thirty minutes a day on most days of the week, accomplished by incorporating short bouts of activity into their daily schedules. Additionally, all subjects were asked to consume a 1,200-calorie diet and attend a weekly educational weight-loss class.

Now there was an interesting concept. It seemed that the study was comparing traditional, structured exercise to something called "lifestyle activity." Participants in this group were not told to start pumping iron or running on a treadmill, but rather to try and squeeze short bouts of activity into their day by doing seemingly minor things such as taking the stairs where possible or walking instead of driving short distances. It sounded good, but could such an exercise strategy really cause an obese person to lose weight? Surely a formal exercise class would be much more effective for losing weight than just bits of exercise done throughout the day.

Well, when all was said and done, here's how things turned out: After sixteen weeks, members of the step-aerobics group lost an average of 18 pounds and members of the lifestyle-activity group lost an average of 17.

Amazed that an *accumulation* of short bouts of activity could be just as beneficial in losing weight as one long stretch of exercise, I looked further into this phenomenon. After all, this was quite the *opposite* of what I had learned. I was always taught that to get the most benefit from exercising, it must be done in one *continuous* session, not broken up into bits and pieces. Further investigation led me to another study:

The International Journal of Obesity published a study of fifty-six overweight women who had been randomly placed into two exercise groups (Jakicic, 1995). One group did a single, long bout of exercise (such as one thirty-minute session a day), while the other did short bouts of exercise (such as one ten-minute session, three times a day). All subjects attended a weekly behavioral weight-control program and were recommended to eat a 1,200- to 1,500-calorie-a-day diet. *After five months, results showed that the subjects in the short-bout group exercised more consistently and lost more weight than those who did one long bout of exercise.*

I was starting to see a definite trend emerging in the literature. But since I prefer not to prescribe a treatment to people based on just a few studies, I kept digging. Here's one last randomized controlled trial I'll tell you about:

A study published in the journal *Metabolism* took thirty-nine men and women who were 15 to 50 pounds overweight and randomized them into either a group doing structured aerobic-exercise activities (stationary cycling, walking on a treadmill, etc., for up to forty-five minutes, three to four days a week) or a lifestyle-activity group (accumulating thirty minutes of moderate-intensity physical activity on most days of the week). All subjects participated in a weekly behavioral group session and were prescribed a self-selected diet of 1,200 to 1,800 calories a day. After three months, *differences in weight loss between the two groups were not significant* (Andersen, 2002).

As my scrutiny of the literature drew to a close, I found more studies, all with similar results. The conclusion from all this research was crystal clear: *It is entirely possible to lose a significant amount of weight by dieting and using an exercise strategy that doesn't involve formal exercise, a big chunk of your time, or special equipment.* In other words, an effective exercise strategy can be whittled down to one simple requirement: Accumulate at least thirty minutes of moderate-intensity activity per day, at least five days of the week.

HERE'S HOW YOU'RE GOING TO LOSE WEIGHT DOING WHAT YOU LIKE TO DO

"Accumulate at least thirty minutes of moderate-intensity activity a day, at least five days of the week." Hmm. Just what exactly does *that* mean?

Essentially, it means that *any* activity in which your body is moving around counts as exercise, but *only* if it is done at a *moderate intensity*. As you can see, what you do isn't nearly as important as how you're doing it—that's because the *intensity* is the key.

If you're not quite sure what moderate-intensity effort is or isn't, don't worry. Here are some of the ways moderate-intensity activity has been described that should give you a good idea:

◆ It's how you feel when you're walking briskly—that is, three to four miles an hour, or the pace at which you walk when you are late to a meeting or doctor's appointment.

◆ You should feel some exertion, but still be able to carry on a conversation comfortably.

◆ You should feel like you're actually doing a little something but not doing it so vigorously that you couldn't keep it up for a little while.

Now that you know what moderate intensity is supposed to feel like, here are some suggestions of things you can do that count toward the thirty minutes of moderate-intensity activity you need to accumulate each day:

Everyday Activities

◆ briskly walking to class, to work, to the store, for pleasure, the dog, as a break from work

◆ mowing or raking the lawn

◆ bagging grass or leaves

◆ hoeing

◆ weeding while standing or bending

◆ planting trees

◆ trimming shrubs or trees

◆ hauling branches

◆ stacking wood

◆ pushing a tiller

◆ shoveling light snow

◆ scrubbing the floor or bathtub while on hands and knees

◆ hanging laundry on a clothesline

- sweeping an indoor area
- cleaning out the garage
- washing windows
- moving light furniture
- packing or unpacking boxes
- carrying heavy bags of trash, recyclables, water, or firewood
- putting groceries away
- actively playing with children (walking, running, climbing)
- pushing a child in a stroller
- pushing an adult in a wheelchair
- bathing and dressing an adult
- feeding farm animals
- actively playing with or training pets
- cleaning gutters
- caulking
- refinishing furniture
- sanding floors with a power sander
- laying or removing carpet or tiles
- roofing
- painting inside or outside your home
- wallpapering
- washing and waxing the car

Fun Activities

- hiking
- roller skating
- bicycling
- juggling
- ballroom, line, square, folk, modern, disco, and ballet dancing
- table tennis
- tennis
- shooting baskets
- playing Frisbee
- playing badminton
- fencing
- downhill skiing
- ice skating
- swimming
- treading water
- water skiing
- snorkeling
- surfing
- canoeing
- kayaking
- saddling or grooming a horse
- skateboarding

The Usual Exercises Can Count Too

◆ aerobics classes

◆ weight lifting

◆ running

◆ stair steppers

◆ elliptical machines

◆ walking

◆ stationary bicycle

◆ exercise videos

(Adapted in part from the CDC website: www.cdc.gov/nccdphp/dnpa/zphysical/pdf/PA_Intensity_table_2_1.pdf)

These are just some suggestions. Remember, any activity can be counted as part of your thirty minutes a day, as long as your body is moving around and it's done at a moderate level of intensity. Although it's not a requirement in any way, shape, or form for you to lose weight, it is certainly okay for you to do more than the thirty minutes of accumulated activity a day and to do it more vigorously. I also recommend that everyone get the go ahead from his or her doctor before starting any kind of exercise program.

HOW TO GET STARTED... TODAY!

I want you to put down this book and try something. We're going to get in a short bout of moderate-intensity exercise right here and now, so get out your watch and keep an eye on it for the next two to three minutes. Take a brisk walk up and down the hall, around your house, or outside. If you can't leave the room, just stand up and march in place, briskly bringing your legs up and down. Got it? See you in a few minutes.

How was that? Were you able to go the whole time? Did you feel like you got the intensity up to a moderate level, that is, where you felt like you were exerting yourself a little, but not so hard that you couldn't carry on a conversation comfortably? If not, don't worry about it. It's perfectly fine to work up to it if you have to. Just remember, the more often you do it, the more your body will get used to it and the better shape you'll be in—putting you just one more step closer to your goals.

The point of all this is to give you an example of just how easy it really is to fit in a short exercise session throughout the day. But don't get me wrong: If you want to lift weights or go running for thirty minutes, that's fantastic and you should go for it; you will certainly meet your minimum exercise requirement for the day!

For a lot of people, though, traditional exercise options just don't work for a variety of reasons we've already talked about. That's the beauty of the "lifestyle" type of exercise. You can turn a lot of activities you *love* to do into beneficial exercise to help you lose weight and stay healthy. With a little thought and planning and such a broad range of exercise options, most *everybody* should be able to incorporate thirty minutes of accumulated exercise into their schedule at least five days a week.

To help you keep track of your daily exercise, I'm going to provide you with a handy card to use (see page 99). As with the calorie-intake cards, a blank copy is included in the back of the book so you can easily make more copies.

Looking at the card, you can see how easy it is to use. Just stick it in your pocket, and every time you complete one minute of moderate-intensity activity, simply check off a box. If your card isn't convenient to use at the moment, just check off the minute later. It's quite alright to estimate if you need to. We're not doing brain surgery here.

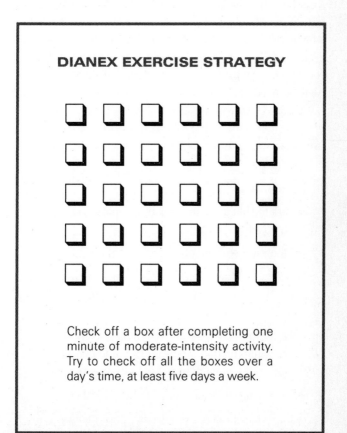

DIANEX EXERCISE STRATEGY

Check off a box after completing one minute of moderate-intensity activity. Try to check off all the boxes over a day's time, at least five days a week.

Although to some readers this may sound like a lot of time to accumulate throughout the day, it really isn't. Let's say you go for a five-minute brisk walk at lunch. Well, go ahead and check off *five* boxes! Add that to a ten-minute brisk walk after dinner, and you're already *half* done with your exercise for the day. Then, try either raking leaves, scrubbing the shower to music, or vacuuming the rug for fifteen minutes, and you can call it a day! See what I mean? The possibilities are practically endless, and remember, this *exact* exercise strategy has already been properly tested and found effective in randomized controlled trials using people who needed to lose a lot of weight. Therefore, you can rest assured that your effort is *not* going to be wasted!

Consider some of the following ways to easily incorporate moderate-intensity activities into your daily schedule:

- Take a two-minute brisk walk during a television commercial.

- Park farther away from your destination so you can get in a brisk walk.

- Don't forget that you can walk at the mall, too.

- Take advantage of outdoor activities, such as mowing the grass with a push mower, weeding, or digging a new garden.

- Household chores you have to do anyway, such as sweeping the floor or cleaning windows or the bathtub, count when done at a moderate intensity.

- Try taking the stairs instead of the elevator.

- Get a treadmill or exercise bike and use it in front of the television.

◆ Walk while the kids are at soccer practice.

◆ Dance to music you enjoy.

One of the goals of this particular exercise strategy is to get you looking at exercise a bit differently than you *ever* have in the past. Instead of thinking that exercise must involve huge chunks of time every day when you're sweating your tail off, change your perspective a bit. Within each day, see the small openings that pop up here and there that could be used to get in a two-minute, five-minute, or ten-minute brisk walk. On days when it's really not possible to squeeze in this kind of traditional exercise, just think of doing the activities you *have* to do with a moderate intensity. According to many randomized controlled trials, all those little opportunities you take advantage of throughout the day add up to one *big* opportunity to lose weight.

Chapter 5 in a Nutshell

◆ Many randomized controlled trials have shown that as long as exercise is done at a moderate intensity, many short exercise sessions done over a day's time are just as effective for losing weight as one long session.

◆ Any activity can be counted as exercise as long as your body is moving around and the activity is done at a moderate level of intensity. Randomized controlled trials have shown that when everyday activities, such as housecleaning or yard work, are done in this manner, they are just as effective in helping you to lose weight as traditional forms of exercise, such as running on a treadmill.

◆ An effective exercise strategy to lose weight is to accumulate at least thirty minutes of moderate-intensity activity every day, at least five days of the week, using either lifestyle activities, traditional exercises, or a combination of the two.

What People Who Successfully Manage Their Weight Have in Common

Success is often reached by doing simple things that others are not doing.

Open up any popular weight-loss book and you'll probably find no shortage of before-and-after pictures. These would be photos of people who have used the information in the book and made amazing transformations.

Now don't misunderstand—there's absolutely nothing wrong with a book sharing its success stories. Just keep one thing in mind when it comes to this type of support for a book's effectiveness: You're only getting *half* the story.

Why only half the story? Well, if you stop and think about it, what you're looking at on the page are pictures of people who have used a particular plan and succeeded in making a positive change—a change most anybody would surely be happy with. The question is, what happened *after* the pictures were taken? Not the next day, mind you, but a little farther on down the road. Were they able to keep their bodies looking like the picture you see in the book for, say, six months? How did they look a year later? I wonder what a snapshot of those same people looked like then.

One would think that if an author had pictures of people looking like a million bucks after being on their plan for several years, they'd be plastered all over the book. Funny how I've never seen a single one of *that* kind of picture.

The bottom line is that most books have no trouble showing you plenty of colorful before-and-after photos, which no doubt help persuade many people to buy the book. That's all fine and good, but what we really need to see are the long-term "after" photos—that is, about a year or two "after." It is only then that we can be sure how a plan holds up over the long run, before a person commits their precious time and effort. After all, who wants to follow a surefire weight-loss plan if it is doable or only works for a matter of months?

Nobody. And herein lies the purpose of this chapter. We're going to take a good look at published studies that have been done on people who have been successful at keeping weight off for a long period of time. Not just individuals who lost weight, mind you, but those who lost it *and* kept it off. By doing this, we will find out not only how they did it, but also what habits they have in common.

As you will soon see, the vast majority of such individuals use the same kind of strategies that you have learned about in this book. I have already proven the Dianex Strategy to be effective, based on numerous randomized controlled trials. Now I'm going to show you research that lends further support to this strategy and also demonstrates that losing weight *and keeping it off* can actually be a very realistic goal.

LITTLE-KNOWN FACTS ABOUT PEOPLE WHO KEEP THE WEIGHT OFF

One way to figure out how to lose weight and keep it off is to simply talk to people who have done it. One could then make a list of all the things these people have in common and put the information to good use. The question is, in order for you to write down general statements about people who successfully manage their weight, how many of them do you think you should talk to? For instance, most would agree that talking to a small number of people, say five, wouldn't be nearly enough to get an accurate picture of things.

But what about talking to twenty individuals? Fifty? Perhaps one hundred would be about right.

This is exactly where I was when I took a look at the research done in this area. Quite obvious was the fact that a great many of these studies made *big* conclusions from talking to only a *small* number of subjects who successfully managed their weight. It was then that I began to wonder if any of the research in this area really meant much at all.

Not one to give up, I continued searching every nook and cranny of the scientific literature to find larger and larger studies. Then one day my luck changed. I came across a study that had been done on people who were members of the National Weight Control Registry. Curious about this registry, I investigated further. Here's what I uncovered:

◆ The National Weight Control Registry was established in 1994 in order to investigate the characteristics and behaviors of people who have lost weight and kept it off.

- ◆ It is the largest ongoing study of successful weight-loss maintainers.

- ◆ To be a member of the registry, you must be at least eighteen years old, have lost at least 30 pounds, and have maintained a loss of at least 30 pounds for one year or longer.

- ◆ The registry currently consists of over three thousand members.

Now this was more like it. *Hundreds* of subjects, all successful at losing weight and keeping it off, just waiting to be researched—and researched they are. To date there have been numerous studies conducted on registry members, a group whose numbers continue to grow each year.

With all of this in mind, it's time to take a brief look at what some of the exciting research has revealed about this group of "successful losers." The information you are about to read has been adapted entirely from two articles that were published in peer-reviewed journals (Klem, 1997; Wing, 2001) unless otherwise noted.

Q: First of all, is it impossible to lose weight if you've been overweight most of your life?

A: Absolutely not. Registry members were very overweight before their successful weight loss. We know this because as a group, they had an average maximum lifetime BMI of 35! Also noteworthy is the fact that about half of them said that they first became overweight by the age of eleven, and 25 percent of them could recall becoming overweight between ages twelve and eighteen.

Q: And their parents—were they overweight?

A: You're right if you guessed yes. A lot of these successful losers did have overweight parents. About half of them said they had one overweight parent, while 27 percent of them said both of their parents were overweight.

Now this is what I call encouraging. Here is a group of *hundreds* of people who were not only very heavy individuals as adults, but as children too, *and* they typically had one or more overweight parents. Still, they managed to find a way to lose weight and keep it off. The next question, of course, is how did they do it?

Q: People who successfully maintain their weight loss—how did they lose it?

A: To begin with, let's talk about help. Do most people who successfully manage their weight lose it on their own, or did they get help from other sources, such as dieticians or Weight Watchers?

Well, approximately 55 percent of registry members lost their weight by getting help. The remaining 45 percent reported that they had lost weight on their own. As you can see, it's almost a fifty-fifty split.

Q: The question of help or no help aside, what methods did they use?

A: Eighty-nine percent of successful losers reported changing both their diet *and* their physical-activity level to lose weight. Interestingly, only 10 percent of registry members changed just their diet to lose weight, and a dinky 1 percent changed just their activity level.

A few more specifics. Of those who *did* modify their diets to lose weight, 88 percent limited their intake of certain types or classes of foods, 44 percent limited the quantity of food that they ate, and 44 percent counted calories. Also, while almost every member of the registry changed their activity level to lose weight, 92 percent reported that they exercised at home, 31 percent exercised with a group, and 40 percent with a friend.

From these results, I think it is quite safe to say that diet and exercise *combined* was the number-one method used to lose weight by this huge group of people successful at maintaining their weight loss. Sound familiar?

Q: People who successfully manage their weight—how do they keep it off?

A: When researchers looked at how registry members *maintained* their weight loss, they found three common strategies: eating a diet low in fat and high in carbohydrates, regular physical activity, and frequent self-monitoring of their weight. Here are some interesting details about each strategy:

- The average registry member consumes about 1,381 calories daily by eating nearly five meals or snacks.

- About 24 percent of those calories come from fat, 19 percent from protein, and 56 percent from carbohydrates. *Less than 1 percent of registry participants consume a low-carbohydrate diet.*

- They eat out about three times a week.

- The strategy most frequently used to limit food intake is to limit eating certain kinds of foods.

- Only 9 percent of registry members are able to maintain their weight loss *without* regular physical activity.

- Over 75 percent of registry members include walking for exercise. Other common activities include cycling, weight lifting, aerobics, running, and stair climbing.

- Thirty-eight percent of registry members weigh themselves daily. Seventy-five percent weigh themselves at least once a week.

I find it very fascinating, especially with the popularity of the low-carbohydrate diet, that less than 1 percent of people successful at losing weight and keeping it off for years actually report using such an approach.

Not so surprising, though, is that they consume a low-calorie diet and regularly exercise.

Q: What triggers successful weight loss?

A: Fact: Before finally succeeding, 90 percent of registry members tried to lose weight but failed.

Hmm. Makes you curious as to what happened that allowed them to finally succeed, doesn't it?

When asked, the majority of the members of the registry said there wasn't really any particular factor they could put their finger on that distinguished this successful weight loss from past attempts, other than noting a greater commitment, much stricter dieting, and an increased role for exercise.

Interesting. It appears as though their eventual success was not due to a revolutionary new diet plan or to starting a sophisticated workout routine. Instead, it seems that they essentially got more committed and motivated than ever before to carry out simple diet and exercise strategies.

This indeed could be the case, because over two-thirds of registry members said there was a "triggering event" or occurrence that came before their successful weight loss. Here are a few of the types of events they mentioned:

- ◆ 32 percent reported a *medical* triggering event (for example, fatigue, varicose veins, sleep apnea, low-back pain)

- ◆ 32 percent reported an *emotional* triggering event (such as their spouse leaving them because they were fat)

- ◆ 4 percent were inspired by someone

- ◆ 3 percent saw themselves in a mirror or a photograph

As you can see, it doesn't really matter if you call them "triggering events" or "motivating factors," which is the term I have used in this book. Just know that the majority of people who successfully manage their weight have one, which seems to make the difference between "trying again" and *finally* succeeding.

Q: Breakfast—to eat or not to eat?

A: Often an issue that comes up when discussing weight loss is whether it is best for people to eat breakfast or just skip it entirely. To find out if eating breakfast is a common characteristic of those who successfully manage their weight, researchers asked 2,959 members of the registry (Wyatt, 2002).

The results were striking. Seventy-eight percent of subjects said they regularly ate breakfast every day of the week, while only 4 percent reported *never* eating breakfast at all. This makes eating breakfast an important factor to consider when trying to manage one's weight.

Q: Keeping the weight off—harder or easier over time?

A: If you're wondering if it will always be an uphill battle to keep your weight off or if it will actually get easier over time, then you'll be very anxious to hear about the results of this particular study (Klem, 2000).

This time, 931 subjects from the registry were divided into three groups based on how long they had maintained their weight loss. The first group had successfully managed their weight for two to three years, the second group for three to six years, and the third for six or more years. The researchers then looked at many different things, one being how much effort the subjects felt they devoted to maintaining their weight. Additionally, subjects were given a checklist of weight-control strategies (such as recording food intake, keeping exercise records, or eating out less) and asked to indicate which ones they had used in the past year. Results showed that those who maintained their weight loss *the longest* had several things in common:

- They used *fewer* weight-maintenance strategies.

- They reported that *less* effort was required to maintain their weight.

In short, these findings suggest that the longer you maintain your weight loss, the less effort it will take and the fewer strategies you will need to keep it there.

THIS IS WHY I KNOW YOU CAN LOSE WEIGHT AND KEEP IT OFF

Whether you realize it or not, in the last few pages you have just read many years' worth of research, done entirely on people who have successfully managed their weight.

While this chapter contains plenty of information and tips that you can readily put to good use, I want to make sure that you leave it with at least one thought in mind: If hundreds of people can lose weight and keep it off, it is truly something that can be done.

Recall that many registry members were overweight as children and continued to be very heavy throughout some portion of their adult life. Heck, a lot of then even had parents who struggled with the very same problem. And luck wasn't exactly on their side either; 90 percent of them had tried to lose weight in the past *and failed*. Yet, despite the odds stacked against them, they managed to get the motivation to put simple diet and exercise strategies to work—verified by the fact that the average registry member has lost 66 pounds and kept it off for five and a half years!

Perhaps the biggest lesson to be learned from the studies of the National Weight Control Registry members is that successfully managing your weight is possible, it can be done, and you can do it.

Chapter 6 in a Nutshell

◆ To get accurate information about people who successfully manage their weight, it is best to talk to as many of these people as possible.

◆ *The National Weight Control Registry* is a good place to get such information. It has more than three thousand members who have lost significant amounts of weight *and* kept it off for long periods of time. Much published research has been done on these registry members.

◆ Many members of the registry were overweight as children.

◆ About half of registry members lost weight without outside assistance, and 89 percent of members used both diet and exercise strategies to lose their weight.

◆ Three common strategies many registry members use to maintain their weight include a low-fat/high-carbohydrate diet, regular physical activity, and frequent self-monitoring of their weight. *Less than 1 percent eat a low-carbohydrate diet.*

◆ Only 9 percent can keep their weight down without regular physical activity.

◆ The average registry member eats nearly five meals or snacks a day and eats out about three times a week. Seventy-eight percent regularly eat breakfast.

◆ Before finally succeeding, 90 percent of registry members tried to lose weight but failed.

◆ Over two-thirds of registry members report a "triggering event" that came before their successful weight loss.

◆ Research findings on registry members suggest that the longer you maintain your weight loss, the less effort it will take, and the fewer strategies you will need to keep it there.

7

How to Get on Target and Stay There

Every road you've ever traveled has a bump or two. The
road to success is no exception.

As you feel the pages between your fingers, you can
tell we're almost to the end of the book. That
means we're all done, right?

Not quite.

What you have just read is not a diet book. It's not an
exercise book either. No, I prefer to think of it as a means to
an end, a book to get you pointed in the right direction.
The rest, as they say, is up to you.

But what will you do now?

HERE'S WHERE YOU NEED TO START

You can buy a lawn mower, but it won't be able to cut a single blade of grass until you give it some fuel. Likewise, you
will be unable to carry out any of the diet or exercise strategies in this book for long until you have some gas to get
you going. What I'm talking about here is *motivation*.

While there is no lab test for motivation, and we have

yet to see it on an X ray, we all know it exists. It's that feeling you have when you're driven to do something, the force that keeps you going until you're totally satisfied the job's done. Motivation is that necessary ingredient in everyone I know who has ever done anything amazing. A person simply could not make it to the top of Mount Everest, run a marathon, or summon the strength to swim the entire English Channel without really, really wanting it.

So the first thing to do after you've finished reading this book is to think about your level of motivation. If it's there, you'll know it, and that means you're good and ready to put the Dianex Strategy into action.

On the other hand, if you aren't fully motivated yet, don't worry. That just means you'll have to do a little bit more searching. Try going back to Chapter 2 and taking another look at my list of motivating factors. You may even want to sit someplace quiet for a while so you can concentrate better. For some, writing things down helps them see a situation more clearly. Whatever works for you, just remember, in order for a motivating factor to be really effective and to last, *it must be meaningful to you and give you something you really want.*

To me, that's the whole key here, and it's also where things often go haywire. So many times people get a temporary burst of motivation. Maybe it's New Year's resolution time, or perhaps a class reunion is coming up. While these most certainly count as motivating factors and are powerful enough to get a lot of people off the couch and eating better, all they usually amount to is a temporary burst that fizzles out over a period of weeks or months. Although the motivation was there, it just wasn't meaningful enough to the person to last very long. On the other hand, the motivating factor that is both truly meaningful and gives you something you really want will provide plenty of gas to keep you going over the long run and beyond.

Above all, don't get discouraged if your motivation is low at this point. I am here to tell you that you definitely are getting there. And how can I be so sure? By the simple fact that you're sitting here right now, this very second, reading this book. That means you are at least thinking about losing weight. The process of change *has already begun*.

NEXT, PUT YOUR MOTIVATION TO GOOD USE

I'd like to think that this book is different from any other book you've *ever* read on losing weight. Here are a few reasons why I hope this is true, but you be the judge.

Whereas most books say they have a proven method of losing weight, I have given you strategies that have been demonstrated to work in multiple randomized controlled trials, the highest form of proof in medicine that a treatment is really effective. Whereas most books show you before-and-after pictures as evidence that their plans work, I have shown you the published research on hundreds of people who have successfully managed their weight *for years* and did so by using strategies similar to those presented in this book. Whereas most books have famous celebrities praising their diet and exercise plans, my endorsements consist of an extensive reference section in the back of the book, filled with scientific studies taken straight from the weight-loss research.

The point of all this? I want you to be able to rest assured that you will not be spinning your wheels when you use the diet and exercise strategies described in this book. Like a lot of people, you're probably already busy enough. You don't need someone coming along and asking you to put what's left of your time and energy into something that may or may not work.

That's why I meticulously go through the scientific literature and then only suggest methods that have been shown to work in controlled trials. Anything less and I risk wasting your time. In this case, I offered you one diet strategy, calculating your calorie needs and keeping track of what you eat with a calorie card, and one exercise strategy, accumulating thirty minutes a day of moderate-intensity activity. Because these strategies are based on solid clinical trials, you can be confident that your motivation will definitely be put to good use when you bring them into play.

Effective weight-loss tools are now at your disposal, perhaps for the first time ever. Start by using the calorie and exercise cards included in the back of this book. If you need a refresher on how to use them, simply refer to the summaries at the ends of Chapters 4 and 5.

TO DEAL WITH BUMPS IN THE ROAD, TRY THIS

While many of my patients have accused me of being optimistic—and it's true that I do usually see the glass as half full—I am realistic as well. No plan, however well thought out, is always going to go by the book. A few snags we can get around, but let's face it, some obstacles are just plain unavoidable. For instance, what would you do if you started implementing the diet and exercise strategies presented in this book, and then three weeks later:

> You get an attack of back pain and can't move around very well,

> *or, perhaps,*

> you lose your job.

Heaven forbid that either of these things happen. However, sooner or later something is bound to come up, be it a big or a small setback. That's just the way life is. As gloomy as this may sound, know that there is something you can do that will help soften the blow of setbacks: Simply *expect* that they will happen now and then.

While you never really know what is going to find you or when it will hit you, it is my opinion, based on my own life experience, observing my patients, and good old common sense, that being mentally prepared puts you one step ahead. It's kind of like the old saying, "Forewarned is forearmed."

When you're caught off guard, a setback has the power to throw you way off your target. Being mentally prepared, on the other hand, can lessen the shock *and* get you back on track much, much faster.

Here is a list of some common setbacks that may someday cross your path and throw a monkey wrench into your ability to stick to your diet and exercise strategies:

- ◆ vacations
- ◆ business trips
- ◆ holidays

- ◆ sickness or injury
- ◆ bad weather
- ◆ busy work schedule
- ◆ caring for a sick person
- ◆ having company
- ◆ relationship difficulties
- ◆ death or sudden illness of a loved one

Because every person's situation is different, and life can take so many unexpected turns, it would be impractical and ineffective for me to list specific strategies for dealing with each of the above setbacks. Doing so would probably require another book devoted entirely to that topic. (In fact, many helpful books do exist that offer methods for coping with these sorts of life challenges.) What's true about dealing with any setback, however, is the benefit that comes from being mentally prepared for one *before* it happens. When you adopt this kind of a mindset, it can definitely be much easier to get back on track when you've momentarily fallen off.

THE MOST IMPORTANT THING TO FOCUS ON

It's a safe bet that you have some kind of goal in mind when it comes to losing weight. Maybe it's to lose twenty pounds. Or perhaps you just want to fit into your old jeans. While I'm convinced that everybody should definitely have goals to keep them on target, sometimes goals can get you into trouble. And when might that happen?

When you either don't meet them fast enough or you set them way too high.

These are common pitfalls that I come across almost every day while working with patients and their health problems. For instance, someone might set a goal of getting out of the hospital by Christmas or getting rid of their back pain by next week. Sometimes these goals work out, sometimes they don't. When they don't work out, it's usually due to either an unrealistic goal or an unrealistic time frame. In the worst cases, the disappointment can be overwhelming, and patients just give up their efforts altogether—totally overlooking the progress they have made and how far they have really come.

That's why I say we should approach things a little bit differently.

First, go ahead and set your goals. Goals are necessary for many reasons and downright essential for keeping your motivation up. But once you've made them, remember this: Keep your goals firmly in mind, *but focus mainly on the progress you're making*. It's so important to acknowledge even the *smallest* steps you take toward your goal. For instance, whether you realize it or not, you've already accomplished one step: You're reading this book! Congratulations! And once you've used a calorie card or an exercise card for even *one* day, take a moment to congratulate yourself because you've taken one more step toward your goal. Before you know it, those small steps will begin to add up to measurable progress—progress you need to remind yourself of when one of those bumps in the road appears out of nowhere.

Looking at things this way can put you in a win-win situation. If you meet your goals, that's great—time to set the next ones. If you don't, but if you've been focusing on your progress, you'll be less likely to give up because you know that progress *is* being made and you *are* still headed in the right direction.

In Closing

Beside my desk, at the hospital where I work, are literally hundreds of medical studies from peer-reviewed journals that I have read over the years, organized by subject in black binders. This is the foundation of my physical-therapy practice and also the source from which I have pulled all the information you have just read in this book. It is my hope that I have pointed you in the right direction by giving you a few no-nonsense tools to help you with your weight-loss goals. Equally important to your success, however, is that "something" that made you first open this book.

Good luck. I've enjoyed sharing this information with you.

References

CHAPTER 1

Gwinup, G., et al., 1971. Thickness of subcutaneous fat and activity of underlying muscles. *Annals of Internal Medicine.* 74: 408–11.

Katch, F., et al., 1984. Effects of sit-up exercise training on adipose cell size and adiposity. *Research Quarterly for Exercise and Sport.* 55: 242–47.

Katz, D., 2002. *The Way To Eat: A Six-Step Path to Lifelong Weight Control.* Naperville, IL: Sourcebooks Trade.

National Institutes of Health, 1998. *Clinical guidelines on the identification, evaluation, and treatment of overweight and obesity in adults.* Bethesda, MD: Department of Health and Human Services, National Institutes of Health, National Heart, Lung, and Blood Institute.

Pi-Sunyer, F. X., 1999. Comorbidities of overweight and obesity: Current evidence and research issues. *Medicine and Science in Sports and Exercise.* 31: S602–8.

Rosenbaum, M., et al., 1998. An exploratory investigation of the morphology and biochemistry of cellulite. *Plastic and Reconstructive Surgery.* 101: 1934–39.

Stunkard, A. J., Wadden, T. A., eds., 1993. *Obesity: Theory and Therapy,* 2nd ed. New York: Raven Press.

CHAPTER 3

Alford, B., et al., 1990. The effects of variations in carbohydrate, protein, and fat content of the diet upon weight loss, blood values, and nutrient intake of adult obese women. *Journal of the American Dietetic Association*. 90: 534–40.

Bloom, W., 1959. Fasting as an introduction to the treatment of obesity. *Metabolism*. 8: 214–20.

Dengel, J., et al., 1995. Effect of an American Heart Association diet, with or without weight loss, on lipids in obese middle-aged and older men. *The American Journal of Clinical Nutrition*. 62: 715–21.

Donnelly, J., et al., 2003. Effects of a sixteen-month randomized controlled exercise trial on body weight and composition in young, overweight men and women: The midwest exercise trial. *Archives of Internal Medicine*. 163: 1343–50.

Fortmann, S., et al., 1988. Effects of weight loss on clinic and ambulatory blood pressure in normotensive men. *The American Journal of Cardiology*. 62: 89–93.

Foster, G., et al., 2003. A randomized trial of a low-carbohydrate diet for obesity. *The New England Journal of Medicine*. 348: 2082–90.

Golay, A., et al., 1996. Similar weight loss with low or high carbohydrate diets. *The American Journal of Clinical Nutrition*. 63: 174–78.

Gordon, N., et al., 1997. Comparison of single versus multiple lifestyle interventions: Are the antihypertensive effects of exercise training and diet-induced weight loss additive? *The American Journal of Cardiology*. 79: 763–67.

Guinness Book of Records, 1971. London: Guinness Superlatives Ltd.

Hagan, R., et al., 1986. The effects of aerobic conditioning and/or caloric restriction in overweight men and women. *Medicine and Science in Sports and Exercise*. 18: 87–94.

Hinkleman, L., et al., 1993. The effects of a walking program on body composition and serum lipids and lipoproteins in overweight women. *The Journal of Sports Medicine and Physical Fitness*. 33: 49–58.

Katzel, L., et al., 1995. Effects of weight loss vs. aerobic exercise training on risk factors for coronary disease in healthy obese, middle-aged, and older men: A randomized controlled trial. *Journal of the American Medical Association*. 274: 1915–21.

King, A., et al., 1991. Group vs. home-based exercise training in healthy older men and women: A community-based clinical trial. *Journal of the American Medical Association*. 266: 1535–42.

Miller, W., et al., 1997. A meta-analysis of the past 25 years of weight-loss research using diet, exercise, or diet plus exercise intervention. *International Journal of Obesity*. 21: 941–47.

National Task Force on the Prevention and Treatment of Obesity, 1993. Very low calorie diets. *Journal of the American Medical Association*. 270: 967–74.

Nieman, D., et al., 2002. Reducing diet and/or exercise training decreases the lipid and lipoprotein risk factors of moderately obese women. *Journal of the American College of Nutrition*. 21: 344–50.

Piatti, P., et al., 1993. Insulin sensitivity and lipid levels in obese subjects after slimming diets with different complex and simple carbohydrate content. *International Journal of Obesity*. 17: 375–81.

Stamler, R., et al., 1987. Nutritional therapy for high blood pressure: Final report of a four-year randomized controlled trial— The hypertension control program. *Journal of the American Medical Association*. 257: 1484–91.

Stewart, W., Fleming, L., 1973. Features of a successful therapeutic fast of 382 days' duration. *Postgraduate Medical Journal*. 49: 203–9.

Utter, A., et al., 2000. Effects of exercise training on gallbladder function in an obese female population. *Medicine and Science in Sports and Exercise*. 32: 41–45.

Wadden, T. A., et al., 1989. Treatment of obesity by very low calorie diet, behavioral therapy, and their combination: A five-year perspective. *International Journal of Obesity*. 13 (suppl. 2): 39–46.

Wadden, T. A., et al., 1990. Long-term effects of dieting on resting metabolic rate in obese outpatients. *Journal of the American Medical Association*. 264: 707–11.

Wadden, T. A., et al., 1994. One-year behavioral treatment of obesity: Comparison of moderate and severe caloric restriction and the effects of weight-maintenance therapy. *Journal of Consulting and Clinical Psychology*. 62: 165–71.

Wing, R. R., et al., 1994. Caloric restriction per se is a significant factor in improvements in glycemic control and insulin sensitivity during weight loss in obese NIDDM patients. *Diabetes Care*. 17: 30–36.

Wood, P., et al., 1988. Changes in plasma lipids and lipoproteins in overweight men during weight loss through dieting as compared with exercise. *The New England Journal of Medicine*. 319: 1173–79.

CHAPTER 4

National Academy of Sciences, 2002. Report brief. Dietary reference intakes for energy, carbohydrate, fiber, fat, fatty acids, cholesterol, protein, and amino acids. http://www.iom.edu/file.asp?id=4154.

Van Way III, Charles, 1992. Variability of the Harris-Benedict equation in recently published textbooks. *Journal of Parenteral and Enteral Nutrition.* 16: 566–68.

For nutrient tables see:
http://www.iom.edu/includes/DBFile.asp?id=7300

CHAPTER 5

Andersen, R., et al., 1999. Effects of lifestyle activity vs. structured aerobic exercise in obese women: A randomized trial. *The Journal of the American Medical Association.* 281: 335–40.

Andersen, R., et al., 2002. Physiologic changes after diet combined with structured aerobic exercise or lifestyle activity. *Metabolism.* 51: 1528–33.

Jakicic, J., et al., 1995. Prescribing exercise in multiple short bouts versus one continuous bout: Effects on adherence, cardiorespiratory fitness, and weight loss in overweight women. *International Journal of Obesity.* 19: 893–901.

CHAPTER 6

Klem, M., et al., 1997. A descriptive study of individuals successful at long-term maintenance of substantial weight loss. *American Journal of Clinical Nutrition.* 66: 239–46.

Klem, M., et al., 2000. Does weight-loss maintenance become easier over time? *Obesity Research.* 8: 438–44.

Wing, R., Hill, J., 2001. Successful weight-loss maintenance. *Annual Review of Nutrition.* 21: 323–41.

Wyatt, H., et al., 2002. Long-term weight loss and breakfast in subjects in the National Weight Control Registry. *Obesity Research.* 10: 78–82.

Blank Calorie-Intake Cards and Exercise Cards

Here are blank cards that you can copy and use for keeping track of your daily calorie intake and minutes of activity. See Chapter 4, pages 55–73, and Chapter 5, pages 90–101, for guidelines on how to use them; these tips are also repeated on the back of the cards.

Su M T W T F Sa (circle one)   Calories per food item

Breakfast _____   _____

_____   _____

_____   _____

_____   _____

_____   _____

                     Total for breakfast   _____

Lunch _____   _____

_____   _____

_____   _____

_____   _____

                        Total for lunch   _____

Dinner _____   _____

_____   _____

_____   _____

_____   _____

_____   _____

_____   _____

                       Total for dinner   _____

Snacks _____   _____

_____   _____

_____   _____

_____   _____

                       Total for snacks   _____

Baseline calorie needs _____ Today's calorie intake   _____

Calorie-Intake Card

CALORIE-INTAKE CARDS

Take a minute or two after each meal to jot down the foods you have just eaten as well as the calorie content from any nutrition labels. If you don't have the number of calories right in front of you, take a few minutes to look them up and write them in later on. At the end of the day, finish by totaling the calories for each individual meal (i.e., breakfast, lunch, etc.), and then, going down the right-hand column, add up the totals from all your meals and snacks to get your total calorie intake for the day.

On pages 59–60 you learned how to figure out your Baseline calorie needs (Harris-Benedict equation times appropriate activity factor). If the number you write on the line labeled "Today's calorie intake" is *more* than your "Baseline calorie needs," that means your body will store the extra calories and you'll be gaining weight. On the other hand, if "Today's calorie intake" is *less* than your "Baseline calorie needs," that means you have successfully created a calorie deficit and have forced your body to use up some of its stored fat—so look forward to losing some weight!

Writing down the foods you have eaten and adding up the calories should take you no more than minutes a day. After a week or two of doing this you will find yourself looking at fewer and fewer nutrition labels. Because we have a tendency to eat many of the same foods over and over, you will soon start to become quite familiar with how many calories there are in the foods you eat regularly.

From *The No-Beach, No-Zone, No-Nonsense Weight-Loss Plan*
© 2005 by Jim Johnson, Inc.
Published by Hunter House Inc., Publishers
Additional cards available free by calling
(800) 266-5592 or from www.hunterhouse.com

DIANEX EXERCISE STRATEGY

☐ ☐ ☐ ☐ ☐ ☐

☐ ☐ ☐ ☐ ☐ ☐

☐ ☐ ☐ ☐ ☐ ☐

☐ ☐ ☐ ☐ ☐ ☐

☐ ☐ ☐ ☐ ☐ ☐

Check off a box after completing one minute of moderate-intensity activity. Try to check off all the boxes over a day's time, at least five days a week.

Here are some ways to incorporate moderate-intensity activities into your daily schedule:

– take a brisk walk during a TV commercial

– park farther away from where you're going

– do household chores at moderate intensity

– take the stairs instead of the elevator

– actively play with children and pets

– play Frisbee … learn to juggle … dance

LIFESTYLE EXERCISE STRATEGY CARD

The card is easy to use. Just stick it in your pocket and, every time you complete one minute of moderate-intensity activity, check off a box. If it isn't convenient to use at the moment, just write it down later. It's quite alright to estimate times.

For a lot of people, traditional exercise options don't work for a variety of reasons. That's the beauty of the "lifestyle" type of exercise. You can turn a lot of activities you love to do into beneficial exercise that will help you lose weight and stay healthy.

Although this may sound like a lot of time to accumulate throughout the day, it really isn't. If you go for a brisk five-minute walk at lunch, go ahead and check off *five* boxes! Add that to a ten-minute brisk walk after dinner, and you've done half your exercise for the day.

Any activity can be counted as part of your thirty minutes a day, as long as your body is moving around and the activity is done at a moderate level of intensity. It is certainly okay for you to do more than thirty minutes of activity a day and to do it more vigorously.

I recommend that everyone get the go ahead from his or her doctor before starting any kind of exercise program.

From *The No-Beach, No-Zone, No-Nonsense Weight-Loss Plan*
© 2005 by Jim Johnson, Inc.
Published by Hunter House Inc., Publishers
Additional cards available free by calling
(800) 266-5592 or from www.hunterhouse.com